I0001040

William Browning, Royal College of Physicians of Edinburgh

The Normal and Pathological Circulation in the Central Nervous System

Original Studies

William Browning, Royal College of Physicians of Edinburgh

The Normal and Pathological Circulation in the Central Nervous System
Original Studies

ISBN/EAN: 9783742820242

Manufactured in Europe, USA, Canada, Australia, Japa

Cover: Foto ©Lupo / pixelio.de

Manufactured and distributed by brebook publishing software
(www.brebook.com)

William Browning, Royal College of Physicians of Edinburgh

The Normal and Pathological Circulation in the Central Nervous System

THE

NORMAL AND PATHOLOGICAL CIRCULATION

IN THE

CENTRAL NERVOUS SYSTEM

(*MYEL-ENCEPHALON*).

ORIGINAL STUDIES

BY

WILLIAM BROWNING, Ph.B., M.D.,

ATTENDING NEUROLOGIST TO THE KINGS COUNTY HOSPITAL, AND CONSULTING TO THE
ST. CHRISTOPHER'S HOSPITAL FOR BABIES; LECTURER ON NORMAL NEUROLOGY AT
THE LONG ISLAND COLLEGE HOSPITAL; MEMBER OF THE BROOKLYN SOCIETY
FOR NEUROLOGY, THE MEDICAL SOCIETY OF THE STATE OF NEW
YORK, THE ASSOCIATION OF AMERICAN ANATOMISTS, AND
THE AMERICAN NEUROLOGICAL ASSOCIATION.

PHILADELPHIA :

J. B. LIPPINCOTT COMPANY.

1897.

COPYRIGHT, 1897,
BY
J. B. LIPPINCOTT COMPANY.

TO THE MEMORY

OF THE LATE

PROFESSOR WILHELM BRAUNE,

OF LEIPSIC,

IN REMEMBRANCE OF HIS INVALUABLE CONTRIBUTIONS IN ANATOMY,
OF HIS EMINENCE AND KINDLY PERSONALITY AS A TEACHER,
AND IN PARTICULAR OF THE INCENTIVE THAT HE GAVE
THE WRITER TO TAKE UP THIS LINE OF WORK,
THESE VERY IMPERFECT CHAPTERS ARE
MOST REVERENTIALLY INSCRIBED.

PREFACE.

WHILE a systematic and comprehensive treatise on the encranial circulation might be more generally acceptable, it is proposed here to give only such special articles as shall embody something of originality. A portion of the work is a reproduction of various scattered papers already published, but which are here used as a basis for further additions.

The first six articles are anatomical and experimental; the remaining take up clinical and pathological topics.

It was intended to include some work on the normal pressure in the dural sinuses, with descriptions of a new plan for measuring the same. But this subject has meanwhile been so fully treated by Hill that anything further thereon seems superfluous at the present time.

It is a pleasure to make acknowledgment of aid from many sources. I must particularize Dr. N. T. Beers for excellent drawings and assistance, Dr. E. G. Zabriskie for aid in most of the experiments, Mr. Stucke for artistic work, Professor J. M. Van Cott and the Hoagland Laboratory, the late Dr. J. A. Arnold, and especially Dr. J. T. Duryea, his successor as superintendent of the Kings County Hospital, besides the kind collaborators.   And more especially am I indebted to Captain Joseph Ware, of New York, for much trouble and expense in supplying monkeys from Mexico for certain of the studies.   Without these animals, together with the facilities of the laboratory and of the hospital so freely placed at my disposal, much of this work would have been impossible.

54 LEFFERTS PLACE, BROOKLYN, May, 1897.

CONTENTS.

I.

AN EXAMINATION OF THE SPINAL EFFERENTS FOR THE CEREBRO-SPINAL FLUID.*

THE question of the ultimate absorbents or points of discharge of the cephalo-rachidian fluid—those by which the fluid finally leaves the cerebro-spinal subarachnoid sac—is a very important one, and considerable work has been done in the direction of answering it. In connection with the subject of hydrocephalus (treated in a subsequent chapter) it became necessary to review our knowledge of the matter. This brought out the fact that, so far as concerns the spinal outlets in man, the present teaching is apparently based on the results obtained in animals, and hence, in reality, inconclusive.

In regard to the strictly cranial outlets, the field has been repeatedly worked over. The studies of Key and Retzius, backed by Quincke, F. Fischer (Waldeyer), Kollman, and others, drew attention to the Pacchionian bodies as important paths of discharge (like overflow taps). Though this view has not met with universal acceptance, and so good an observer as Trolard (1892) decides positively against it, the evidence† in its favor is very strong. The great increase

---

* Read before the Association of American Anatomists at the Washington meeting, May 5, 1897.

† Reiner and Schnitzler's experiments with the absorption of ferrocyanide of potash and also of oil from the subarachnoid space (Wien, 1894, *v. Neurlgc. Cntbl.*, 1895, p. 19) showed that it reached the venous current within the skull. Their supposed stomata may as well be the Pacchionian absorbents.

of these bodies in adult life has militated against this theory. But the results to be described in this paper offer a better understanding of the relation.

More certain efferents are the sheaths of outgoing cranial nerves. Along the optic the space extends to the bulbus. Connections of this kind have been shown with the cellular tissue in the nasal cavity. And other similar paths have been described. The proof that absorption by these routes actually occurs was furnished not only by injections on the cadaver but also by the special deposits of suspended particles injected in animals.

The recent claims by L. Hill, of a more general filtration off of the fluid, can hardly apply to conditions as we meet them in practice.

In any case the tendency of the fluid in bipeds is to sink by gravity into the spinal sac, and from there find some way out, even if it has to do this by returning again to the cranial cavity. The effect of gravity on the position of this fluid was long since shown by Luschka ("Adergeflechte d. Mensch. Gehirns," 1855, p. 73).

Most of the published studies on the absorption of this fluid in man have been devoted to the cranial efferents. Possibly previous workers have not caught the clue that is afforded by the change in the human from fœtal to postnatal conditions. There is, then, the more reason for extending our knowledge of this subject as regards the spinal efferents, and it is wholly to this phase of the question that the present experiments have been devoted.

My injections of the spinal subarachnoid space have usually been made from the cervical or top-dorsal region, and, of course, directed caudad. The material used has been either the customary solution of Prussian blue or

Loeffler's aqueous alkaline solution of methyl blue, suitably diluted. It is necessary to employ a liquid with distinguishable color, and yet free from floating particles. Various degrees of pressure have been exerted, but a moderate force accomplishes quite as much as more, and is less open to criticism.

The following description is based on the results obtained by a series of injections practised on the bodies of two monkeys and one cat, on four fœtal subjects, and on the cadavers of six humans ranging in age from a month-old infant all the way up to nearly seventy years.

IN ANIMALS.

As monkeys are partly bipeds, they offer the best analogy to man in this respect also. In their upright position gravity sends the fluid down the spine by preference. Both these animals were full-grown, though young and healthy. The one was supposed to be about thirteen months and the other sixteen months old when used. The injections were made while the body was still warm, and hence before the possible interference of post-mortem changes,—a better guarantee of natural conditions than can often be secured in the human. With each, after removal of the head, the inverted trunk was hung up long enough to empty the vertebral canal as much as possible of all fluids.

As in neither did the injection pass out beyond the root ganglia along any of the costal—i.e., proximal—nerves, it is clear that any moderate pressure used did not force false passages.

This was further shown in the one positive case by the gradually lessening depth of color along the cord, away

from the point of injection. Section of the roots showed
the color in the surrounding sheath only.

In one of these animals—the one, too, where the greater
pressure was used, and where the material passed more
completely down to the termination of the arachnoid sac
in the cauda equina—the color did not at any point extend
out beyond the root ganglia.

In the case of the other (younger) monkey the findings
were, for the most part, the same. Only at one point was
there anything calling for further mention. On following
out peripherally the large lumbars one pair of nerves (the
third lumbar?) was found, each of which showed the following : Well beyond the ganglion and quite outside the
vertebræ, on the upper side of (cephalad) but not surrounding the nerve, was a little blue pouch. The two were the
same in appearance, were equidistant from the cord, and
each extended along the nerve about one-half centimetre.
The channel by which the solution had reached this was
not discovered, though it was, doubtless, along the nerve-
sheath. The distance from the point of injection, together
with the considerable obstruction and but moderate pressure used, must have prevented the forcing of any false
passage. Moreover, the symmetrical arrangement of these
small spaces precluded any suspicion of artefact. Here
was an extra-vertebral extension or connection of the regular subarachnoid space, evidently an outlet for cerebro-
spinal fluid.

As the younger animal even did not show as ample
spinal exits as either dogs or the human fœtus, while the
older one failed to show any at all, it is easy to conclude
that in them the spinal efferents were in the stage of closing
up. The monkey seems to correspond partly to man,

representing an intermediary course between him and lower animals. At the same stage in the individual monkey's development these passages are only less completely closed than in the human.

In the case of a large two-year-old cat the injection failed to pass very freely down the whole length of the cord. Yet it did run out along the third lumbar nerve for a short distance into the muscles at the back of the abdominal cavity.

Quincke ("Zur Physiologie der Cerebrospinalflüssigkeit," reprinted from *Dubois-Reymond's Archiv*, 1872), from experimental injection of cinnabar-emulsion into the spinal subarachnoid space of living dogs, found that "In several cases the cinnabar could be followed on the lumbar nerves to the region of the lumbar plexus between the origins of the psoas, as well as in the sciatic plexus beyond its entrance into the pelvis."

And Key and Retzius (*Arch. f. Mikroskop. Anat.*, 1873, Bd. ix.), in Fig. 39, picture the injection of the sacro-lumbar plexus from the spinal subarachnoid in the dog.

IN THE HUMAN.

The subjects of post-natal age covered the whole period of life, and were essayed in the following order :

1. Female of about sixty-eight years ; dead of dysentery.

2. Female of forty-nine years ; erysipelas and pulmonary sequel.

3. Female of twenty-six years ; syphilitic disease in pons.

4. Male child of six months.

5. Male infant of two months and ten days ; marasmus.

6. Female infant of premature birth, that had lived twenty-four days.

Of course, only unfrozen cadavers are of use, and the fresher the better. With the exception of the two youngest subjects, the findings in the series were so uniform that one description covers all.

On incising the arachnoid there was always an outflow of free, clear fluid. Its discharge was assisted by temporary inversion, leaving a collapsed sheath. This last appears to become more fully distended to a wide canal in old subjects.

Each was injected from the cervical region. The ample filling of the space all the way down showed that sufficient pressure had been transmitted to all parts. The whole cordon of roots on each side was then exposed. These showed the blue color as far as the root ganglia, but never and at no point beyond. Sometimes the nerves at the back of the abdominal and pleural cavities were first examined before cutting away the vertebral arches, but the findings were the same.

The root ganglion was never blued to any extent, and only on its central side. On the anterior root, as specially noted by Dr. Beers, the color did not extend quite as fully or far peripherally as on the posterior,—the limitation of each taken together constituting an oblique line.

The result in the subject of two months and ten days differed but slightly from that in the older ones as just outlined. Several drops of clear fluid ran off on incising the arachnoid. It was injected from the mid-dorsal region. No blue was found anywhere by tracing up the nerves centripetally to the vertebræ. And on following out the roots from the cord the color was found to go, as usual, just to the root ganglia, except along two corresponding roots on each side,—the first and second lumbars. These all showed the same condition. The posterior roots, barely as far as the ganglia, were fully blued as usual. Each anterior root, however, showed a couple of distinct but rather fine blue lines, reaching by and about three millimetres beyond the termination of the ganglion. The blue in each stopped just there. Hence, evidently, a little stump of the fœtal absorbent was not yet obliterated.

The youngest subject of this series was an infant born at about the seventh month of pregnancy, and that had lived twenty-four days (weight, two and three-fourths pounds ; at birth, three pounds). Used thirteen hours post-mortem. Here again injection showed but slight difference from the adult. No free fluid on opening the spinal arachnoid.

The right ileo-hypogastric nerve showed on its ventral aspect a single distinct, slightly sinuous blue line, quite like a minute vessel, that extended about one centimetre peripherally from the root ganglion and came down the anterior root. The anterior crural roots (middle and upper primary trunks) on each side were more or less blue in the surrounding sheaths to just beyond the exit from the vertebral column, but not farther.

As this infant had not reached the usual age at birth (from time of conception), and yet had lived some weeks, the findings are interesting. The outlets had become almost, though not quite fully, closed up. This indicates that the obliterating process is a natural result of post-uterine living.

IN THE FŒTUS.

There were four subjects from this period, corresponding to the sixth and seventh months of pregnancy, respectively, —not, of course, including the premature infant described last above. The results of these fœtal injections were so similar to each other that they also can be summarized together. In each the outcome was positive. For first study of. the whole cord the injection was made from the cervical region. But, to obtain the best results, the cannula in two was inserted in the dorsal region.

The appearance of the nerves above the lumbars (*i.e.*, of the dorsals and cervicals) was the same as in all the post-natal subjects. There was no extension of the material along these beyond the root ganglia, and neither was there any bluing of the nerves from the extremity of the cord, including the sciatics.

The direction of the efferents was found to be invariably towards the abdominal cavity. The roots and trunk of the anterior crural nerve are the main paths, and along these the material may pass well down into the pelvis. In one case the nerves that follow around the flank (ileo-hypogastric, etc.) had participated. In one there was considerable diffuse bluing of the psoas muscle towards its insertion (indicating that the material had escaped from any direct arachno-spinal extensions), in this respect corresponding to an observation on the dog above cited.

Not even in these fœtal examples have the sciatics ever shown any injection, though in animals such a result has been described.

DISCUSSION.

My results, taken together with the facts previously known, lead to a very definite conclusion, and one with which they all harmonize completely.

Outlets for the cerebro-spinal fluid exist along the lumbar nerves in the lower animals at all ages, but in the human only during fœtal or uterine life. The monkey may represent an intermediary.

This wide difference between animal and living human conditions, as well as between fœtal and post-natal in man, does not appear to have ever been recognized.

Numerous points that call for discussion immediately suggest themselves, and can in part be answered here.

1. Are these nerve-sheath extensions of the spinal sub-arachnoid space real exits for the fluid?

This is shown with reasonable certainty by the results of simple injection.

It has further been repeatedly shown by a scattering of the injected material in the upper part of the psoas muscle (for the dog, by previous workers; in the human fœtus, by my own injection).

It is again proven by the special deposit here of sus-pended material injected about the cord. Of course, the result of such experiments applies to all cases where the passages are otherwise known to exist, even though it is only possible to carry them out on an animal.

That a minimal amount of absorption may occur per the parietes of the spinal sac itself is possible, but it cannot be material.

2. At what time does this obliteration of the spinal exits in man occur?

It has not begun up to birth, and yet is practically com-plete by the time the infant is two and a half months old. In fact, this result is, reasoning from the case of premature birth, probably reached in full-term cases by the end of the first month, and even earlier. My cases show that this transition is not an instantaneous process, but one that it takes a little time to complete. It must begin very shortly after if not directly from birth, and constitutes one of the earliest changes of extra-uterine life.

2

There may well be some individual difference in this regard. Though there is no evidence of persistent remains
of this sort, it would be strange if such never occurred.

3. How is this obliteration effected, and to what agencies
is it due?

From the observations in animals, my partial result in
the monkey, my positive in the fœtal, but negative in older
human subjects, it is apparently demonstrated that the upright position in man is the main factor in shutting off the
lower or spinal absorbents.

It may be objected to this that these efferents close up
in early infancy, and hence before the upright position has
been to any extent assumed. So far as concerns the immediate mechanism of closure, this may be true. But it
is explained by the corresponding fact that, while all the
lower animals, old or young, rest and sleep on their bellies,
the human infant sleeps and lives altogether on its back,
or at most but slightly over on its side,—a reversal of the
conditions of intra-abdominal pressure. Very likely this
change in pressure about the lines of exit plays the important part. The result in the infant of two months shows
that the primary closure of the exits is not as far up as is
the final, and this indicates some agency ventrad of the
spinal column.

Or there may be other and less mechanical morpho-
logical factors at work.

In the place of the spinal efferents the arachnoidal villi
and, perhaps, the other cranial outlets increase as life ad-
vances and afford adequate substitutes.

It is worth noting that these spinal efferents apparently
run out chiefly along the anterior roots, and that as they
close up we, for a time, find as temporary remnants certain

fine passages that have all the appearance of distinct vessels. Finally these also disappear.

4. This knowledge helps to explain a number of matters.
It presumably has some bearing on the occurrence of lumbar spina bifida, and on the frequent development of hydrocephalus after its removal.* It throws the onus of the
congenital form of hydrocephalus on the lumbar region ; it
harmonizes with the increase of arachnoidal villi in adult
life ; it shows how the cushion of arachnoidal fluid about
the cord, at the base of the brain, etc., is supported,—*i.e.*,
prevented from leaking off. As this last is a very important safeguard or protector of the brain in man, we see how
essential a factor in the change of body-position to the upright must be this coördinate or preliminary closing up of
the spinal outlets.

This free column of water about the cord in the adult
means a considerable hydrostatic pressure on the lower
spinal structures, approximately a pound to the square inch

---

* An interesting point is the possible purpose of such arachnoceles as occur
in spina bifida, meningocele, traumatic hydrencephalocele, etc. That such
pouches serve as special absorbent diverticula for the fluid is suggested by
various facts.

Not rarely a spina bifida is accompanied by some hydrocephalus. Or
often the removal of such a tumor is followed by the development of resp.
an increase of a hydrocephalus.

Similarly with the cranial forms, there are cases like the following : A small
meningocele just at the base of the occiput was removed successfully from a
child some time after birth. Directly thereafter hydrocephalus began to develop, of which previously there had been no evidence.

Now, it is not probable that the operative or cicatricial contraction shuts off
the normal discharge, since in the spinal type, at least, there are no longer
important local absorbents to be affected. But if their walls can absorb, then
it is clear that their removal might have such effect. This also makes it ex-
plicable why hydrencephaloceles sometimes show a tendency to shrink,—this
occurring if other and more natural outlets develop.

in an average male when upright. The daily recumbency of sleep goes far towards delaying untoward consequences. While the healthy and vigorous may experience no effects therefrom, in the feeble and senile the finer nutrition of the yielding structures of the lower cord and its roots may indeed suffer. This suggests itself as one cause for certain cases of senile paraplegia, in which the upper extremities are fairly intact.

[Despite the ample material available, it has not been possible to secure a full-term fœtus for this purpose. To that extent this line of investigation is as yet unavoidably incomplete.]

II.

THE CHEMICAL IDENTIFICATION OF CEREBRO-SPINAL FLUID.[*]

THE cerebro-spinal fluid differs from other serous fluids in chemical composition to such an extent that it may be differentiated from them by simple chemical tests. This fluid ought to be regarded as a true secretion rather than as an exudate.

The fluid, when pathologically increased in quantity, does not usually depart from the normal composition. After tapping a sac filled with cerebro-spinal fluid a number of times there is apt to be some inflammatory exudate (or transudation), which partakes of the properties of other serous or inflammatory exudates. Cerebro-spinal fluid contains but traces of serum albumin, the proteids being usually in the form of albumoses.

There is usually present no fibrinogen ; hence, this fluid does not clot.

All the proteids of cerebro-spinal fluid are precipitable by saturating the solution with magnesium sulphate. Serum albumin is not precipitated by this salt, and hence must be absent.

Sometimes there is found a specimen which gives a small

---

[*] By Elias H. Bartley, B.S., M.D., Professor of Chemistry at the Long Island College Hospital, from his paper in the *Journal of Nervous and Mental Disease* for 1893.

amount of serum albumin coagulum on boiling. The albumoses are precipitated by cold nitric acid, but the coagulum dissolves on warming, to reappear on cooling.

The specific gravity of cerebro-spinal fluid is generally lower than that of other serous fluids. It ranges from 1005 to 1010. The albumoses, like peptones, give the biuret reaction, or pink color, with Fehling's solution. Cerebro-spinal fluid reduces Fehling's solution, owing to the presence of a substance believed to be pyrocatechin.

To apply these facts to the practical examination of a suspected fluid we may proceed as follows :

1. Boil, when there should be not more than a trace of coagulum of serum globulin and serum albumin.

2. Cold nitric acid ought to form a precipitate, which disappears on heating, and separates again on cooling.

3. Saturation with magnesium sulphate should give a precipitate. Saturation with sodium chloride should also produce a precipitate. Ammonium sulphate may be tried, if the above salts fail.

4. The solution floated upon Fehling's solution should give a pink or rose-red zone at the line of contact.

5. When boiled with Fehling's solution, there should be a reduction of the copper—pyrocatechin.

6. The specific gravity should be between 1005 and 1010.

In repeated tappings, the later ones give inflammatory products with serum albumin, together with the albumoses, —*i.e.*, they coagulate with heat and nitric acid.

III.

As these animals are so important, both for experimental and comparative study, it is desirable to have a thorough knowledge of their encranial circulation. So far as concerns the arteries, the field has been repeatedly traversed. Through the courtesy of the author I have had Rojecki's work for comparison ("Sur la Circulation artérielle chez le Macacus cynomolgus et le Macacus sinicus," reprinted from *Jrnl. de l'Anatomie*, 1891).

On the venous side special descriptions seem to be wanting. The chief subject used for this study was a full-grown male Mexican monkey (*Ateles geoffroii*). At the instance of Dr. Van Cott the following plan was adopted to free the head-vessels as much as possible from blood, and so avoid the formation of obstructing clots.

The animal was chloroformed; both carotids were exposed while yet pulsating, and ligatures loosely adjusted. The one on the left was tied, a slit cut in the vessel just cephalad, and a cannula bound in. While normal salt solution was injected through this, the right carotid was tied and severed just above. By this means there was a free back-flow from the latter vessel, and the internal carotid system was supplied wholly with salt solution. Were it not for the lesser vertebrals this method would soon exsanguinate the whole brain. As it was, the con-

23

dition found on exposing that organ showed that the plan had succeeded well so far as concerned the carotid distribution.

After death of the animal the head was removed, right carotid clamped, vessels further washed out, and for a brief period the alinjection of Wilder practised. Permanent injection of the veins some hours later.

The following description is based principally on this specimen, though a second brain, injected centrally, was also used to decide some features more fully :

1. On cutting away the scalp two small symmetrical venous foramina were noted in occipital bone near median line.

2. No emissaria Santorini found in parietal bones, nor did any appear when injecting later.

3. Length of denuded skull, three and one-fourth inches ; breadth, two and one-half inches.

4. Moderate amount of diploe, and sutures everywhere firmly united.

5. The anterior lobes were much paler than the occipital, the latter still showing some blood in the veins. This difference was, of course, due to the saline solution injected into the carotid (*Vide supra*).

6. Torcular opened. Cannula inserted forward in long sinus, and colored starch solution injected (after cutting away calvarium with ronguer, but with dura otherwise intact). The superior veins filled promptly and well, as could be seen through the transparent dura.

7. The straight sinus was found to empty directly at the torcular, though a slight fold of dura turned the current wholly into the right lateral. The long sinus connected with both laterals, but also turned principally into the

right. In the second specimen, however, the long sinus turned more into the left lateral and the straight sinus into the right.

8. To fill the ventricular veins, my old plan was employed (*v.* "Veins of Brain," pp. 44, 45). After cutting away the skull-cap and loosening the dura, but before taking out the brain, the head is inverted. The internal vessels are thus relieved of all compression. Starch solution is then injected through the sinus rectus. This suspension, together with the washing out *intra vitam* with normal solution, constitutes a very perfect experimental method of injecting the central vessels of the brain. Where such a scheme can be carried out entire success is assured.

9. Foramen of Magendie freely open.

SUPRA-CEREBRAL VEINS. (Plate I., Fig. 1.)

There was a noticeable grouping of these vessels into an anterior set composed of four pairs, and a posterior of four or five pairs. On the right this was more apparent than real, as was shown on drawing away the falx. A like grouping occurs in man.

Those of the anterior set are scattered along some distance apart, while the posterior ones are at their mouths much more bunched.

There is no indication on either side of a so-called vena anastomotica magna. This term was applied by Trolard to a supra-cerebral often larger than the others, and that seemed to offer a special communication between the middle of the longitudinal sinus above and veins in the Sylvian region emptying below. The writer has pointed out, however, that little importance can be attached to this vessel even in man.

The supra-cerebrals from the frontal region show a trifling turn backward just as they near the sinus, thus agreeing with their course in man and most animals. Those more posteriorly, however, turn, *vice versa*, slightly forward on approaching the sinus, yet to a decidedly less extent than they do in the human.

OTHER SUPERFICIAL VEINS.

1. On the left three veins, and on the right two, jumped from the lower border of the occipital lobe to join the lateral sinus.

2. On each side a large vein was seen to reach the dura by leaving the tip or frontal border of the first temporal convolution. This vessel then ran directly outward, under the dura, along the bony crest (sphenoid wing), and straight through the skull into the temporal region just back of the upper level of the orbit. (*v.* Plate II., Fig. 3.) It originated from surface vessels of the temporal lobe. The injection could be followed to the outside of the skull, and without any diminution in the size of the vessel. This shows it to be a true emissary, and one that in the monkey drains a considerable portion of the temporal lobe.

There is often in the human a partial counterpart to this. A considerable vein from the temporal lobe, and sometimes a partner from the adjacent portion of the frontal, either passes under the sphenoid wing to reach the cavernous sinus (as has been supposed), or more rarely runs in the dura around under the temporal lobe, across the whole middle fossa, to reach the supra-petrosal sinus.

The orifice by which this vessel in the monkey leaves the skull, and which is essentially for its transit, is certainly not the "Foramen orbito-temporale der amerikanischen

Affen" described by De Filippi in 1865. And with equal certainty it is not the emissarium temporale * of Luschka. In fact, it does not seem to have been specially recognized, and may fairly be called new. As this opening is through the sphenoid ala to the external temporal fossa, it may be in order to suggest the term "Foramen spheno-temporale" as a proper characterization.

3. The cranial dura runs down between the orbitæ to connect directly with the tissue of the nose. The sinus injection went in a fine stream as far as the cranial limit, and evidently had slight connections through this foramen cæcum.

4. There was no trace of an infra-longitudinal sinus in either specimen (infrequent even in man). But instead there was a large azygos supra-callosal vein. This could be followed two-thirds of the way along the dorsum of the callosum in the median line, ending, as does the smaller vein in man, posteriorly in the vena Galeni. This received numerous branches on either side, running up to the marginal fissure and connecting more or less freely with the descending median branches of the supra-cerebral veins (also like the same in man).

---

* As E. Loewenstein puts it in his thesis ("Ueber das Foramen jugulare spurium und den Canalis temporalis am Schädel des Menschen und einiger Affen," Königsberg, 1895), "The canalis temporalis is during the embryonic period the way by which, through connection with the sinus transversus and the sinus petroso-squamosus, the blood is carried from the skull to the external jugular vein." He found some remaining trace of this foramen jugulare spurium on one side or the other in hardly one out of ten human skulls.

In monkeys he found that, of the Catarrhines, it was not present in nine Cercopithecus skulls, in six Cynocephalus, nor in three Semnopithecus, but could be made out in eleven Inuus ; of the Platyrrhines, it was regularly present in three Ateles skulls, in five Cebus, in three Mycetes, and in four Hafale. He sums up that in this respect the monkey resembles man.

5. A large internal occipital vein also helped to form the group that mass in Galen's vein. It came from the calcarine fissure and adjacent region, all the way forward to the branches of the callosal vein just described.

CŒLIAN VEINS. (Plate I., Fig. 2.)

On cutting fully through the callosum and separating the hemispheres the two cœlian veins (one in each lateral ventricle) were seen to take a lyre-shaped course, uniting beneath the splenium to form the common vein of Galen.

This latter vessel curved upward around the splenium much as in the human subject, only that it made a less acute angle with the sinus rectus. In fact, it entered this at barely a right angle, instead of doubling on itself at this point as in man. Just before emptying it received on its upper or concave aspect the supra-callosal vein already described.

The general arrangement of the ventricular veins, even to the choroidal (double on the right, at least), was practically identical with that in man. The extra-ventricular efferents of Galen's vein represent a slightly more extensive area than in the human.

VEINS OF THE BASE.

On each side there was in both specimens a large vena basilaris. This took the usual branches on the base, including all those deep in the Sylvian fissure. Here, as commonly in the human, there was a wide deviation from the descriptions of our anatomies. The superficial veins of the middle and lower Sylvian region took a course quite distinct from those at the bottom of the fissure. This deep Sylvian to the basilar receives, of course, the small pre-perforating veinules ; but it also extends out beyond them, and at least connects with, if it does not more fully drain, those of the insula. Such a matter is of some import, for, as shown elsewhere, the veins assume new relations much more slowly than do the arteries.

Each basilar emptied centrally, the left into the cœlian vein (velar or intima) near its termination, the right directly into Galen's vein. In man this discharge of the basilar per Galen's vein holds for only about one-half the cases.

As to the floccular and cerebellar veins, it can only be said that in one specimen there was on the right a large vessel coming up along the crus cerebri, directly from the floccular region, to join the basilar vein. This took up *en route* a vein from the fissura hippocampi.

Taken as a whole, the arrangement of the brain-veins in the monkey, while corresponding closely to that in the human, is simpler, shows a more uniform symmetry, and has a more favorable discharge. There is much less counter-delivery to the current on entering the sinuses, in particular as regards Galen's and the post-supra-cerebral veins. The anastomoses, though less marked, are doubtless proportionately large.

In several places, notably over the occipital region towards the long sinus, and also in the lateral ventricles, it was not unusual to find the veins directly cross each other. In places one vein even sent a complete loop directly under another.

IV.

ON THE REMAINS OF A FORAMEN SPHENO-TEMPORALE IN MAN.

In the last paper this name (spheno-temporal foramen or canal) was given to a passage through the great wing of the sphenoid, of some importance to the venous circulation in the brain of the monkey. It is natural to inquire whether something of the kind does not occur occasionally in man also. And examination serves to confirm this supposition.

In a second monkey's skull this vein from the temporal lobe was found to run, on each side, a slightly greater distance along or under the border of the spheno-orbital crest (boundary between middle and anterior cranial fossæ) before passing out through the skull-wall. But its course and destination were essentially as in the first.

In both man and the monkey this foramen or canal passes out through the great wing of the sphenoid. Exteriorly it is analogous to one of the favorite exits for the vena diploctica temporalis anterior, which vessel may empty into the vena temporalis profunda (at the bottom of the external temporal fossa) or may discharge into the sinus alæ parvæ (within the cranium).

Without doubt in the monkey this vein from the temporal lobe, while traversing the diploe, does connect with its vessels.

The fact that this opening lets out a diploic vein may have obscured the other fact that it also serves for the

30

transit of an emissary. This transmitted vein offers a direct communication, more or less frequent in man, between the deep temporal veins and those of the brain proper.

An examination of thirty human skulls (several of them Indian and prehistoric *) from the collection of the Long Island College Hospital was made to determine the constancy of such exits on the outer or temporal surface of the great wing of the sphenoid. Of these thirty there were four with no openings on either side, six with none on the right, and one with none on the left. Hence of the sixty sphenoid alæ forty-five (or seventy-five per cent.) presented such apertures. Even in the negative cases some had substitute openings outward, just under the base of the wing, or apparently by orifices in the neighboring bones.

These openings are usually very small (the largest was barely two millimetres in diameter), and are often two or more in number on each wing. Their most typical location is about the middle of this exterior sphenoid surface. In fifteen (or one-third) it is specially noted that they were about this site ; in nine they were distinctly high or low on the surface ; and in twenty-one this point was not noted (not classifiable).

It is probable, as indicated, that these openings, when present, regularly connect with intracranial vessels. In only two was so straight a passage found that a fine probe could be dropped through into the cranial cavity. In seven others, water injected at the outer orifice flowed through into the inside. In most of the others the opening was too small for practical injection. In all the certain cases the inner orifice was in the anterior wall of the sphenoid

---

* In these the positive results were slightly under the general average.

fossa, under the spheno-orbital crest, and hence, in life, opposite the tip of the temporal lobe. At this point or region on the inner surface are commonly a number of small openings in the bone, giving it a perforate appearance. Here is also a point where, according to many anatomists, the medidural and diploic veins connect quite constantly.

Hence we have here a minor venous confluence,—the pretemporal diploic vein, the medidural vein, and the sphenoidal sinus (in the monkey the vein from the temporal lobe) connecting more or less freely.

The thickness and cancellated structure of the bone at the junction of the sphenoid wing and the angle of the frontal bone serve frequently to obscure and scatter the directness of this communication in the human skull.

In man this passage must connect through the sphenoidal with the cavernous sinus; or instead it may run to the occasionally present inferior sphenoidal sinus of Bell (present, according to Knott, in about twenty-five per cent. of all cases).

Not rarely in man a medicerebral vein (*v.* "Veins of Brain," p. 38) empties into the sphenoidal sinus, and is then analogous to the usual course of the vein in the monkey.

This passage can best be classed as an emissarium of the type inconstant, though common in man. It should be added to such lists as that given by the writer in Buck's "Reference Hand-Book" (vol. viii. p. 243). In the human it is of theoretical rather than practical interest, though it may serve as a minor substitute outlet in thrombosis of the deeper sinuses, or, on rare occasions, be of some importance pathologically in transmitting morbid processes from without.

V.

THE ARRANGEMENT OF THE SUPRA-CEREBRAL VEINS IN MAN, AS BEARING ON THE THEORY OF A DEVELOP-MENTAL ROTATION OF THE BRAIN.*

ALTHOUGH this theory of Alex. Hill was first proposed in 1885, and further elaborated in 1887 (*Brain*, Part 36), the short sketch appended to his translation of Obersteiner (1890) will doubtless serve to gain for it much more general attention. As it has not, however, been worked out much beyond the stage of an attractive suggestion, it may be in order to point out any other facts bearing thereon. In the first place, his view is hardly described in sufficient detail to make it in all respects clear, and at best should not be taken too literally as regards minor points. He compares the form of the perfected mammalian brain, meaning, of course, each hemicerebrum, to that of a ram's horn or of a loop or kink. It might quite as well be likened to one turn of a spiral. To comprehend this more clearly, as applied to the brain, we should remember that a structure may simply enlarge without otherwise changing its internal or external relations, or it may, without change in volume, undergo any variation in shape ; or, finally, as is the view in the present case, it may both enlarge in vol-

---

* Read before the Association of American Anatomists at the Washington Congress, September 24, 1891, and reprinted from the *Journal of Nervous and Mental Disease*, November, 1891.

ume and double or become twisted on itself. That the
human cerebrum, as compared with that of lower orders,
has expanded in certain parts and directions is, of course,
an old observation. But, besides this, the claim is now
made that the primarily straight brain has in its growth
become reflected and curved on itself in such a way that
it may be likened in general outline to a ram's horn, the
apex of the temporal lobe representing the tip of the
horn.

For the present purpose it is not necessary to enter into
the particulars of the theory or the arguments advanced,
further than to say that he makes no use of local circulatory
peculiarities in support of his position.

For instance, the distribution of the precerebral artery
is very suggestive of a reflected field. This is noticeable
in a general way in Duret's plates (*Arch. de Physiolog.*,
Paris, 1874), but is more strikingly apparent in my later ones
(Wood's "Reference Hand-Book," vol. viii., New York,
1889). As these last were simply drawn to fact without
thought of theory, they offer the better evidence. It is
also noticeable, in dissecting out these precerebral branches,
that they run in juxtaposition to the parent stem for a surprising distance before glancing off to their respective
fields.

But it is evident that the arteries, since they are more
under the influence of an internal directing pressure, would
more rapidly conform and adapt themselves to any new
position than would the veins with their interior pressure
almost *nil.* Hence, from the veins, if from either, might
we most naturally expect evidence relating to this point;
and of the veins, those that from this theory would be
subjected to the greatest displacement,—viz., the supra-

cerebrals. These lie along part of the greater curvature of this supposed spiral.

Except very casually, Hill does not consider whether, in this transformation, any rôle is played by the enveloping membranes. However, the pia, being so abundantly connected with the brain by innumerable arterioles and veinules, and also so involved by folds in the fissures, must naturally be carried along to the same extent as the apposed cerebral tissue. The more external membranes, on the contrary, are but slightly connected with the brain, and as in any such twisting of the brain its envelopes must naturally, for their own part, perform a purely passive rôle, it follows that the dura and skull are not carried along *in toto*, but simply conform by expansion or contraction to the growth-demands of the subjacent brain proper. Hence, at the only points, exclusive of the base, where there are any connections between dura and pia, some results of the tension produced by the dragging of the one on the other would be probable. The main connections of this kind are again the supra-cerebral veins.

On this point part of the evidence to be quoted was published a full year before the first appearance of Hill's proposition, and hence may safely be considered free from any bias of previous knowledge. ("Veins of the Brain," Brooklyn, 1884, pp. 14, 15): "It was long since observed that the more anterior supra-cerebrals take a course very nearly at right angles to the sinus, and that the posterior ones take more and more an oblique course, to such an extent that the most posterior ones must run forward a distance of three to four centimetres. Here they terminate in the sinus, with a very acute angle, against the blood-current. The vein coming from the convexity makes

at the edge of the longitudinal fissure, or somewhat farther
out and back in the pia, the necessary angle in order to
approach the sinus as described.   It then runs a short distance forward before leaving the pia. . . . The anterior
supra-cerebrals, more often than the posterior ones, spring
over from the pia to the dura at some distance (one to
three or four centimetres) laterally from the sinus.*

"The posterior ones reach the side of the sinus, and the
most posterior ones even curve forward before leaving the
pia, but the distance from this point to that where they
empty into the sinus is at least equal to that in the varying
anterior ones." Page 15 : "The anterior (supra-cerebral)
veins empty above or at the side of the sinus, comparatively unhindered, as though they came straight from the
dura.   The veins farther back, however, discharge more
and more at the side and bottom of the sinus, and those
farthest back empty almost without exception at the bottom.   Many of the latter, indeed, must take an upward
course through the falx cerebri and travel a considerable
distance before they reach the lowest part of the sinus."
On this last matter Trolard had previously made a similar
observation.   The above quotations sufficiently indicate the
facts which, it is believed, have some relation to the rotation theory.

Page 54 : "*Development.* If one bears in mind that
the brain in its growth doubles, so to speak, over backward
and elongates somewhat, it is easy to see that from this . . .
the brain would carry the pia, with its veins, backward,—
the posterior ones a considerable distance, the anterior ones

---

* This further progressive distinction between the anterior and the posterior
supra-cerebrals has since been again and more fully studied by Mittenzweig,
(1889).

little or none at all." (Foot-note.) "This can be prettily illustrated with a column of soft potter's clay. A stout cord runs straight along one side from end to end, representing the sinus longitudinalis ; small cross-strings firmly fastened to the large one at equal distances, a little pressed into the clay, but with their ends free, represent the supra-cerebrals. If now we fix one end of the column and cord, and then bend the other end of the column in a direction away from the cord, the latter will be seen to no longer reach the whole length of the now convex side ; while of the cross-strings, the first are about as before, —rectangular to the sinus ; those farther back have been so pulled forward and down that they can be followed some distance beside the main cord before they pass out around the column. This corresponds closely to what seems to have occurred in man."

Page 55: "The appearance on one small fœtal brain tended to substantiate this,—*i.e.*, the posterior veins did not stand so oblique to the sinus as in the brains of adults." This is very conclusively shown by the illustrations in the more recent work of E. Hédon ("Étude Anatomique sur la Circulation Veineuse de l'Encéphale," Paris, 1888). Plate V., Fig, 1, from a human fœtus of three and a half months, shows no indication of this angular attitude of the posterior supra-cerebral veins. Plate V., Fig. 2, from a fœtus of six and a half or seven months, gives some evidence of this arrangement, whilst in Plate VI., Fig. E, the usual position of these veins in the human adult is outlined and can be compared with the immature forms.

If it were possible to determine the proper size of column, calculations or experiments might be made with it and the results compared with measurements from a number of adult human brains *in situ*, with a view to determine mathematically how far the argument from the veins bears out the theory.

Further, it is probable that the closing up in fœtal, or at latest during infantile, life of the prolongation of the longitudinal sinus through the foramen cæcum may be explained by the same retracting action of the supra-cerebrals at their junction with the said sinus, especially as the maximum tension, so far as the sinus line is concerned, would be exerted at this point.

Although the evidence from the vascular arrangements as here cited only applies to a portion of the cerebrum, it at least so far corroborates the rotatory or spiral theory, or adds interest to it as a working theory.

VI.

ON THE EXPERIMENTAL DETERMINATION OF THE METHOD OF DEVELOPMENT OF SYMMETRICAL BRAIN-HEMORRHAGES.

In a later chapter, in connection with the subject of bilateral cerebral hemorrhages, the following question arises : Does the influence producing these effusions emanate from some common centre, as in the pons, or is the one focus primary and the other induced in consequence? It is quite possible to imagine such an influence, transmitted by commissural fibres of the callosum.

And, first, can this be answered by experiment? If it be but an occasional occurrence dependent on peculiar and unusual conditions, then we might not be able to satisfy the requirements. Otherwise a general principle is involved, and it ought to be possible to settle this experimentally.

Direct observation of any place on the brain, corresponding to some translateral point stimulated, must be futile. The effects of the necessary exposure to air, of the anæsthetic employed (stupefying consciousness and hence cortical functions), or if no analgesic be employed, then the altered cortical innervation due to fright and pain must rob any such attempt of all claims to exactness. If, perchance, it should succeed, well and good, but failure would be indecisive.

39

Another and more promising plan is to produce, artificially, a focus, with as little other injury as possible. Then let the animal come fully out from the influence of any anæsthetic used, and continue under as normal conditions as possible for any desired period. Finally, examine the corresponding parts on the non-operated side for any signs of change.

In pursuance of this plan the following experiment was performed. As only one was done on the monkey and one on the dog, any conclusions drawn from them are subject to revisal.

A healthy, vigorous Mexican monkey was operated as follows : Chloroform anæsthesia. A short incision was made over the right parietal region, and a fine hole bored through the skull,—scant two centimetres from the median line. Then a sharp, flat-pointed needle was inserted vertically a limited distance into the hemisphere, and the tip twirled around eccentrically for the purpose of tearing up tissue and making a hemorrhagic focus in the middle of the centrum semiovale. On coming out of the anæsthetic the animal was for a time hemiplegic on the left, but he presently recovered fully. At least he appeared to have good use of all extremities, grabbed with both hands, and was active as usual.

Two hours were allowed for the development of any translateral changes, when he was given a lethal amount of chloroform.

The point where the needle entered the cortex was just in front (two to three millimetres) of the middle of the central fissure. The line of puncture could be followed down almost to the ventricle. The main focus was in the albalis immediately above the roof of the cœle. A little leaking had occurred into the ventricle itself. The whole volume of effusion and torn-up tissue, however, was only about the size of a large pea, and not as ample as desired.

Section and examination of corresponding parts on the left failed to show any hemorrhage or definite change. A couple of small vessels in the vicinity were possibly a little fuller than in the neighboring parts ; but, as a whole, the result must be classed as negative.

Whether a larger focus, free of all leaking, and a longer interval between its production and the final examination, would give any positive find must be left undecided for the present.

Another experiment—on the dog—was similar in all respects, including time allowed, and absolutely negative in result.

In the case of the lower animals, it is open to question whether their cranial vaso-motor arrangements correspond sufficiently to those in man to make any experiment of this kind worth considering. Even in the monkey the work will only be decisive when positive results of some kind are obtained. So long as they are merely negative the possibility remains that there is a finer differentiation of these functions in man, and that it cannot be solved by animal experimentation, but by clinical inference.

VII.

A CASE OF INTERNAL HYDROCEPHALUS, DUE TO DISEASE (THROMBOTIC) IN THE WALL OF THE STRAIGHT SINUS.*

THE causes of internal hydrocephalus, exclusive of the forms due to intra-ventricular inflammation and compression of the venous discharge by tumors, are little known. A case which would ordinarily be called idiopathic, but in which a sufficient cause was found, is therefore worth recording. It occurred in a six-year-old girl of German parentage. The first symptoms of the trouble began three months previously : these it is only necessary to state briefly. She had been apparently well until attacked by vomiting. This was followed by convulsive attacks, and later by a variety of indefinite symptoms ; opisthotonus in the convulsive seizures, pain across the forehead or in one or the other ear, general weakness, etc. No paralysis, no trouble with vision, intelligence clear to the last.

She died under the charge of Dr. H. P. Bender, with whom I made the autopsy, and to whom I am indebted for the above notes.

The skull was thick and firm. Brain surface and envelopes healthy except as to the sinuses. No trace of meningitis on either base or convexity. On removing the brain, clear fluid broke through the posterior perforated space.

---

* Reprinted from the *Journal of Nervous and Mental Disease*, April, 1887.
42

The whole amount of fluid was estimated to have been five to six ounces. The superficial gyri were but very moderately flattened. Examination of the ventricles showed the velum interpositum firm and rather thick. No adhesion or other sign of inflammation in the ventricles. Both lateral chambers, and the third and fourth ventricles with the connecting iter, were dilated. The only noticeable alteration in their walls was the dilatation of the veins, especially in their finer branches. This was apparent on the ventricular roof as well as floor (most of the roof-veins discharge through the vena Galeni). The two venæ cerebræ internæ were very broad and contained liquid blood. No cause for the trouble then was discovered in the distended cavities. On examining the sinus rectus, a dark thickened spot immediately attracted attention. This was about half an inch from the anterior end. Starting from the torcular a director readily passed up the sinus until this point was reached, where an obstruction was met. On slitting up the sinus, it was found that opposite the thickening an oblique thin membranous septum had retarded the sound. After opening, it was not possible to say whether the membrane had completely closed the narrowed sinus, the sound having made an opening, or whether a fine slit through it had existed. Immediately adjoining this were several fine fibres crossing from wall to wall, but not like the bands so often seen in the various sinuses. The above-mentioned thickening in the sinus wall affected each side and was in the substance of the wall itself. On cutting through either side, a layer of reddish-gray organized material was found just in the position of the parasinual spaces which occur, in adults at least, even along the straight sinus. This deposit extended about one-third of an inch, the remainder of the sinus being free. The longitudinal sinus showed a somewhat similar though less advanced condition. Its main channel was everywhere free, but the sini subalterni shone through full and black and to the feel presented firm cords. On opening these, a dark fibrinous material, partly organized, was found firmly attached to the surroundings. Here, evidently, a process had been going on quite similar to that beside the straight sinus, but of a more recent date. Moreover, lying below the vessel's channel these thromboses did not materially contract it.

The apex of the right lung was adherent and very hyperæmic, though not presenting any discoverable tubercles.

We know from many cases of cerebellar tumor that compression of the venous discharge from the ventricles may cause internal hydrocephalus. In this case the obstruction developed in the main efferent vessel itself, and hence was not quite parallel, since certain anastomoses may have remained free. As I have elsewhere shown ("Veins of the Brain," 1884), the ventricular veins are terminal vessels, their only connection with other veins— except by the sinus rectus—being in their posterior portion just before uniting. Here certain basilar veins, usually discharging through the vena Galeni, communicate in a roundabout way with other cerebral veins. This limited anastomosis was doubtless but slightly interfered with, except secondarily by the increased pressure from the accumulating fluid.

No history of syphilitic taint or other cause for the peculiar thrombotic condition could be found.

VIII.

A CASE OF INTERNAL HYDROCEPHALUS FROM COMPRES-
SION OF THE VENA GALENI BY A TUBERCULAR EN-
LARGEMENT OF THE CONARIUM (PINEAL GLAND).

GIRL of four and a half years. German parentage.
Never a vigorous child, though of good size for her age.
The present trouble was of about three weeks' duration,
running under the clinical appearance of a meningitis, and
ending in coma. There had been no pupillary symptoms
(normal reactions) and no paralysis.

Autopsy through the courtesy of the attending physician,
Dr. H. P. Bender, March 6, 1891 (thirty-six hours p. m.);
to him are also due the clinical notes already given.

Dura much injected, apparently venous. Small Pacchionian granulations on either side of the longitudinal sinus,
along the line of the incoming cerebral veins. No subdural
adhesions. No old clots in falciform or lateral sinuses.
The brain appeared large ; gyres not noticeably flattened ;
general injection of cortex.

On lifting the brain from the posterior fossa a considerable quantity of clear fluid suddenly appeared,—not, however, more than one or two ounces. This was thought to
have come from the paracœles.

No purulent material anywhere on the surface. A slight
opacity of the arachnoid, where stretched out as over the
Sylvian fossæ or at the base, may have been of post-mortem

origin. Possibly a minute tubercle beside the basilar artery.

The paracœles (lateral ventricles) appeared to have been dilated, and still contained an ounce or so of fluid ; the parietal veins of these cœles were well filled with blood. Epicœle normal in appearance.

The main alteration, in addition to the hydrocephalus, was an enlargement of the pineal gland. This was the size of a small hazel-nut. The little tumor corresponded to the otherwise absent conarium.

The small mass was directly adherent to the vena Galeni, but rested in a bed of yellowish lymph-material directly pressing from above upon the cerebellum (supra-vermis or central lobule). This was in position to compress Galen's vein, and perhaps, also, any lymph-passages from the paracœles. To this mechanical action the moderate hydrocephalus was doubtless due. So far as the cursory examination could establish, it is quite possible that some more general distribution of tubercles in the pia did exist, and the clinical history, with the fatal termination, rather indicated the same.

According to Henoch ("Diseases of Children," New York, 1882), "Experience teaches that tubercles situated in the middle lobe of the cerebellum, or between it and the tentorium, are especially apt to produce effusion into the ventricles from pressure upon the vena magna Galeni and its chief branches."

The marked increase of Pacchionian granulations in cases of cerebro-spinal meningitis was noted by Frölich in 1881 (*Wiener Klinik*).

IX.

A CASE OF TRAUMATIC CEPHALHYDROCELE.*

THE comparative rarity of this trouble, at least of published reports, and some interesting questions involved, suggest that the subject may be worth considering, even though little new can be added.

My case is that of a girl of seven years, seen in October, 1892, a patient of Dr. George E. Law. Her trouble dates from an injury when a year old. The mother, with the child in her arms, fell on the stairs, throwing the girl somewhat violently into a corner. This was immediately followed by convulsions and by left hemiplegia not involving the face. There was no previous paralysis or other abnormity. The physician then in attendance said that the soft cranium had been dented in. At first the head was greatly swollen, and for years a large lump remained over the region of injury. This, however, gradually subsided, so that for the last three years it only puffs out on crying.

A year ago last summer she was in convulsions all one night, and she had another seizure October 7, this year. She has, however, also been having of late so-called faint-

---

* Paper read before the Brooklyn Society for Neurology, November 9, 1892. Here reprinted, with an illustration and other additions, from the *Journal of Nervous and Mental Disease*, 1893, p. 155.

ing spells two or three times a day, and has been less bright
mentally since the first convulsions. The latter are severer
on the left side ; no initial symptom, but a moan ; always of
late yawning and tired ; never complains of headache, unless sometimes of local tenderness on the head from crying ;
the left hemiplegia has very gradually improved, so that
only a paresis remains ; shortening of left extremities
stated ; knee and radial jerks stronger on left than on
right ; left hand cooler than right. For years the left
thumb and fingers were drawn in and the hand was a little
flexed ; but even then, although not possible when awake,
yet in sleep the arm would be freely put up over the head
(*i.e.*, mimic or so-called automatic actions intact,—by some
classed as a thalamic function). Walks limpingly on left
leg ; can just about stand alone on left foot.

Pupils equal ; no distinct hippus. Vision in left eye
possibly impaired, yet fairly good ; in right, normal.
Pulse, 108 (standing). Sleeps well and without special
dreaming. She is a plump, healthy, and bright-looking
child. Cannot read yet, but can count some. Has a lively
interest in everything, is properly inquisitive, laughs, plays,
etc.

There is a long, somewhat transverse depression in the
skull, reaching slightly backward to the left of the median
line, and crossing the sagittal suture an inch or so in front
of the lambdoid. The main part runs from this point
obliquely forward and somewhat downward over the upper
parietal region on the right. The hair-growth and color of
skin over this part are normal. When the child is mentally
excited there is a filling up of the depression ; that, however, can be very easily forced back by pressure with the
finger-tips. It also fills some on compressing the jugulars.

No distinct opening can, however, be felt, though there is evidently one at the bottom of the hollow. When she lies down the whole depression fills up, even a trifle more than level, yet is also very easily emptied, showing a pretty free communication with the encranium.

Pulsation did not seem noticeable when the cyst filled by lowering the head, but became very evident when in erect postures it filled by any mental effort,—*i.e.*, there was decided pulsation only when the fluid was driven up by an actively increased arterial supply to the brain. Perhaps this is the explanation of the fact that in some cases pulsation is observed and in others not, although the size of the communication must also be a factor,—a minute opening diminishing the pulsatory movement.

We aspirated and removed about two drachms of a clear, colorless fluid like water, except for some minute floating particles or shreds. The puncture, through a firm cyst wall, did not appear to cause any pain, nor did the withdrawal of this small quantity of fluid have any perceptible effect on the patient. The cavity immediately refilled, and even leaked some through the oblique puncture while she remained reclining, thus showing an abundant source. Microscopical examination of the aspirated fluid showed : occasionally a leucocyte ; rare irregular flakes and fibres, sometimes a little pigmented ; otherwise only uncertain and foreign matters. Subsequent puncturing failed to do any great amount of good.

Though the total experience with this form of trouble is limited, it suffices to indicate that the cyst in this case connects with the lateral ventricle, and that the fluid is cerebrospinal. Further and decisive proof was given by the chemical examination. This was made by Dr. Bartley,

4

and, as it involves recent methods not (so far as I am aware) ever applied to one of these cases, I have asked him to contribute a brief account of the main decisive tests (*v.* special article, p. 21).

His results in this case were as follows :

Specific gravity (by weight), 1010.

No precipitation by heat.

All proteids precipitated by magnesium sulphate.

A precipitation by cold nitric acid.

No precipitation by hot nitric acid.

With Fehling's solution doubtful.

This excludes serum albumin, but includes albumose, and in general shows that the fluid corresponds well to cerebrospinal, but not to that from any independent cyst.

The differential diagnosis in well-marked cases is almost alone from venous cysts (*v.* Martin, " Venous Blood Tumors of the Cranium," *Journal Am. Medical Association,* September 18 and 25, and October 2, 1886). Hernia cerebri, encephalocele, etc., are often congenital and not readily reducible. Aspiration (and, if necessary, an examination of the fluid) settles the diagnosis.

It has been noted that all cases are in the young. It is not probable that they all die before advancing far in years, but that, as in Southam's case (though in Makins's the opposite was occurring), either the external part shrinks up or the cranial opening becomes shut off spontaneously or by the natural bone-growth, thus leaving simply an encranial cyst (ventricular diverticle), a course that the present case also is following. Evidently of this nature are many of the cases of late glibly dubbed porencephalus : that of Dr. Barber (described at the same meeting), that of Brush, and others. This makes the pathology somewhat comparable to that in cases of syringomyelia starting from the central canal.

As to treatment : One negative indication has been established, both by theory and experience. Do not attempt surgical interference. The cases so far operated appear all to have ended fatally, except that of Halley. Tapping also proves of little use, except when necessary to relieve pressure.

The literature of the subject is not great, the principal English and American papers being,—

R. Clement Lucas : Two cases, each illustrated. *Guy's Hospital Reports*, 1876, 1878, and 1880–81.

Connor : *Am. Journal of Med. Sciences*, July, 1884. He collected twenty-two cases, including two of his own.

Southam : Description accompanied by drawing of case. *Brit. Med. Journal*, May 12, 1888, pp. 1004, 1005.

Makins : *Trans. Clin. Society*, London, 1887, pp. 203, 204.

Halley, of Kansas City : *Jrnl. Am. Med. Assoc.*, 1893, ii. 86, 87. One of his cases (Bertha Thalin) was clearly of this type, and eventually recovered from operation,— probably the first to do so.

My recollection also includes a misplaced society report, probably American.

A few considerations may be added as to the way such cysts (or diverticles of the ventricle) originate. It is at least improbable that a simple rupture of the ventricular wall (ependyma) could alone lead to this result, although it doubtless occurs as a preliminary factor. The case is practically a special form of internal hydrocephalus. There is no evidence to show that this is here kept up by any continuous inflammation of the secreting choroidal villi. There seem to be two possible ways left, involving an interference with either : (*a*) the ventricular venous efferents, or (*b*) the normal discharge of the ventricular fluid. In at least many of these cephalhydrocele cases the connection with the ventricle is at a point in the region of what may be termed the ventricular outlet, or neck of the cœle (in ours, evidently the roof over this part). A slight dragging, displacement, cicatricial constriction, or even fibrinous plugging at this point, might suffice. Until some more exact explanation can be given, I think we may contentedly conclude that obstruction at this outlet is the cause. The same holds also for quite a proportion of the miscellaneous cases of hydrocephalus. Surgical measures, by any plan so far proposed, must prove unavailing in all such cases, largely by reason that the real cause is not removed, and the like applies to all attempts at cure by tapping.

Re-examined December 27, 1896. Condition continues essentially as when first seen. For a couple of years in the interim she was free from convulsions, but an attack of scarlet fever brought them back again. Since the few aspirations in 1892, there has been no swelling of the head over the cleft ; but it still fills up to the edges of bone when she lies down, and then distinct fluctuation can be made out. The fissure is wide and deep in its middle part, with an especially abrupt frontal border. The opening through the skull can be pretty certainly detected an inch or so to the right of the median line.

Is not as forgetful as formerly. Front part of left half of tongue is much atrophied. Sensations of touch and pain are good over left hand ; this part is small and somewhat contracted in fingers and wrist, though more useful than before.

At this time Mr. Stucke kindly made the accompanying sketch. (Plate II., Fig. 4.) It is from direct measurements, and self-explanatory,—the dot representing the midpoint between glabella and occipital protuberance.

X.

LUMBAR PUNCTURE FOR THE REMOVAL OF CEREBRO-SPINAL FLUID.*

THERE are a variety of troubles attended by an increased intracranial pressure, and this often reaches such a degree that relief is imperatively demanded. Brain-tumors, meningitis, hydrocephalus, and, perhaps, some traumatic conditions come under this head ; and the list might include further disorders if some harmless way of relieving were available. Of course, a radical cure by removal of the cause is the true desideratum, but in this class of cases such permanent relief is rarely attainable. Hence we turn to any measure that can give even temporary amelioration. And this seems to be all that can be justly claimed for the method here to be considered.

In a paper on Hydrocephalus, read before the Tenth German Medical Congress (April, 1891), Quincke described the results obtained by puncturing with a hollow needle and allowing the excess of fluid to run off. This he had practised in part by boring fine holes through the skull. But he also described and endorsed a method of introducing such a needle in the lumbar region directly through the skin, between the vertebral arches, and tapping the

---

* Read before the American Neurological Association, Washington, May 31, 1894, and reprinted from the *Journal of Nervous and Mental Disease*, October, 1894.

lumbar subarachnoid space. As the point chosen is below the cord, no serious injury can occur ; at most a puncturing of some nerve or small vessel, perhaps. In an adult he had thus in an hour drawn off eighty centimetres of fluid. He recommended this plan for every hydrocephalus with pressure symptoms, especially in the acute forms, whether simply serous or of tubercular origin. He also suggested subcutaneous slitting of the spinal dura. And this has been done by Parkin—in the lower cervical region, however—as well as practically by others ; yet even this more thorough plan gave but transient relief.

Several others have reported experience with the trocar-method, Von Ziemssen, perhaps, being its most enthusiastic advocate. My first trial was made a year since. As the results have not been very encouraging, I have done it in but few cases. In one—that of an old hydrocephalus with some exacerbation—there was subjective relief. It was also done in two cases of spinal trouble with evidence of compression of the cord. In one of these (traumatic Pott's disease, corroborated by autopsy), it was with a view to possible relief of the distressing jactation, but to no purpose. In the other, where the trouble had developed suddenly after pleurisy, the puncture was for diagnosis, and at least excluded meningeal hemorrhage.

One case may be worth relating more in detail. This and one other were in the service of Dr. Bogart at the M. E. Hospital, and it was through his courtesy that I operated.

Boy of eight months, with gradually increasing hydrocephalus. External strabismus on right. Is apparently blind, though pupils react. Fontanelle large and full and approaching sutures open. Some tonic contracture of legs and arms. As he had first developed an irregular fever and some vomiting, it was a question about proceeding, but we decided that interference was all the more warranted. No anæsthetic. The child alternately slept and cried a little during the withdrawal of an ounce and a quarter. The fontanelle gradually sank in and the sutures closed up, except when the child cried. It was noticed that compression of the head (manual) increased the flow.

Extremities—contracture not relaxed. The child's condition was apparently not influenced by the operation. Temperature as before puncture went at times to 105°. He gradually grew worse, became comatose, and died five days later. The fontanelle had not refilled. Autopsy by Dr. Jelliffe. General congestion of the membranes, with whitish, irregular patches over either temporal apex. Vast clear hydrocephalus of lateral ventricles. It extended freely into the third, and by a short dilated aqueduct into the fourth. This showed a subarachnoid continuation down spine. On opening over the lumbar cord much free clear fluid was found. No apparent injury from the puncture. The appearance suggested that some of the fluid had escaped through the opening and collected in the extra-dural space.

This was a valuable case. At the time of puncture there seemed to be an acute increase of the hydrocephalus, perhaps a developing meningitis. The fact that pressure on the skull accelerated the outflow, that the fontanelle sank and remained so, and that at the autopsy the fourth ventricle was found to participate and the fluid here to connect with that below,—all this shows that the tapping as such was successful. Thus it was a specially favorable case, because of the good evidence that the pressure of the effusion actually was reduced. And yet the intervention did nothing, either to prolong life or relieve symptoms. In many cases, symptomatically like this, the effusion does not extend into the fourth ventricle even, and then there can be little chance of withdrawing fluid from the cerebral collection through any spinal puncture. The entire failure to relieve in this instance has deterred me from performing it in subsequent cases of the kind.

ACCIDENT.

In one case, a girl of twelve years, with a supposed internal hydrocephalus from old meningitis, after only half a drachm had been secured, the respiration stopped. Narcosis was of course discontinued, and, thanks to the prolonged efforts of the staff, the girl was resuscitated. Possibly a very slight elevation of the head, in the hope of increasing the scant flow, may have favored this occurrence ; certainly neither the puncture nor the small quantity withdrawn was thought at all responsible.

DIRECTIONS.

Patient in the recumbent posture on the left side. The knees may be drawn up and the spine flexed, giving a curve posteriorly.

An anæsthetic is usually advisable in adults and older children where normal sensation exists. Still, in these cases with increased brain-pressure there may be more than the usual risk.

Elevating the head has not increased the outflow, and, especially if an anæsthetic be used, is not without danger.

Strict asepsis, needle sterilized, etc.

Usually it is easier to go in between the third and fourth lumbar vertebræ. Only once have I succeeded between the fourth and fifth.

A long, firm, smooth aspirating needle (No. 3 French, or from 2½ to 4) answers well. This can easily be connected with a tube for determining pressure if desired. Special needles have been devised, but seem unnecessary.

Enter a little to one side of the median line (five to ten millimetres laterally, though in children it may be better to pass directly between the spinous processes). As these latter here incline downward, the tip of the needle on reaching the space selected may be tilted up a little the more readily to enter between.

In my adult cases the length inserted, to the opening in the needle, has varied little from five centimetres. In children of eight months and twelve years, respectively, it was only two and a half centimetres. These two figures give about the range of variation (Quincke says from two to six centimetres).

The amount to be drawn off is clearly indicated in each case. It may be allowed to run, or more commonly drip, until the flow spontaneously reduces or ceases. This shows that the pressure is relieved, and yet only within proper limits. There seems to be no danger of air entering. Sometimes the fluid at first comes out tinged with blood collected by the tube in transit, but this then soon gives way to clear, colorless fluid. One case has been reported with turbid fluid from meningeal inflammation, and in one evidence of hemorrhage (intracranial) was found.

No special precautions are necessary on withdrawing the tube or in subsequently treating the puncture (iodoform-collodion, if desired).

It is proper, of course, for the patient to lie quiet for a time.

CONCLUSIONS.

1. The method is simple, easily practised, and rather attractive.

2. In itself it is usually without danger.

3. By it we certainly can draw off cerebro-spinal fluid.

4. The quantity in an adult at short sittings has been from one to one and a half ounces.

5. This, without doubt, represents the amount of free

fluid usually present in the lower vertebral canal, even when occluded above.

6. In internal hydrocephalus the relief, if any, is but very temporary. In the common form due to tubercular meningitis the result is not worth the trouble, while in the closed or sacculated forms it must rather do harm than good.

7. As a diagnostic means—*e.g.*, in suspected meningeal hemorrhage—it is valuable. And as an index of pressure it may also be worth noting.

8. It is worth further trial : (*a*) as a passing relief in brain-tumors not complicated with hydrocephalus ; (*b*) as a substitute for trephining in progressive dementia ; (*c*) in certain spinal troubles ; (*d*) and possibly as a means of applying medication directly to the spinal meninges.

9. In conclusion, it may be said that while admissible in all cases of brain-pressure, there is nevertheless as yet no established indication for this procedure, except for diagnostic purposes.

LITERATURE.

1. II. Quincke.   Ueber Hydrocephalus.   *Verhandlungen d. X. Congr. f. Innere Med.*, 1891.

2. II. Quincke.   Die Lumbalpunction bei Hydrocephalus.   *Berliner klin. Wochnschr.*, 1891.   Nos. 38 and 39.

3. E. Wynter.   Four Cases of Tubercular Meningitis in which Paracentesis of the Theca Vertebralis was performed for the Relief of Fluid-Pressure. *Lancet*, May 2, 1891.

4. O. Wyss.   Zur Therapie des Hydrocephalus.   *Corresp.-Blatt f. Schweizer Aerzte*, 1893.   No. 8.

5. Parkin.   [Opened vertebral canal for relief of fluid-pressure ; case ended fatally.]   *Lancet*, 1893, ii.

6. Von Ziemssen and others.   XII. German Med. Congress.

P. S.—The later foreign literature is too ample for specification here.

Since the publication of the above paper the subject has received considerable attention in this country also, and several articles have appeared.

7. Aug. Caillé, *N. Y. Med. Jrnl.*, June 15, 1895, pp. 750, 751.
8. G. W. Jacoby, *ibid.*, 1895, ii., and 1896, i.
9. D. L. Wolfstein, *Arch. Pediatr.*, March, 1896, pp. 180–191.
10. O. G. T. Kiliani, *N. Y. Med. Jrnl.*, March 14, 1896.
11. W. L. Babcock, *State Hospitals Bulletin*, July, 1896.
12. A. H. Wentworth, *Bost. M. and S. Jrnl.*, Aug. 6 and 13, 1896.
   (Also *Arch. Pediatr.*, Aug., 1896, pp. 567–590.)
13. Caillé, *Arch. Pediatr.*, Aug., 1896, pp. 561–566.
14. C. G. Jennings [case], *ibid.*, p. 591.
15. Wentworth, *Bost. M. and S. J.*, 1897, i. p. 107.

XI.

A CONSIDERATION OF OBSTRUCTIVE HYDROCEPHALUS AND OF THE MECHANICAL PRINCIPLES UPON WHICH ITS DEVELOPMENT DEPENDS.

WHILE there may be little radically new to be said on this subject, certain explanations or theories that have met with but limited acceptance can now be placed on a surer footing, and it is possible to apply more directly than has been done various facts of recent knowledge. No one seems as yet to have undertaken any really comprehensive description of the many points that go to make up the subject. The better the matter is understood, the more certain does it become that all cases of internal hydrocephalus are of this class. Such terms as primary and secondary become consequently obsolete, as applied to hydrocephalus. There is no such thing as primary in any sense in which the term has here been used ; all cases are secondary, or more properly sequelæ.

The classification into acute and chronic forms is an essentially clinical one, and from that point of view justifiable. It,-however, has no significance in the mechanical sense, although a larger proportion of the acute cases than of the chronic may prove to be due to extra-ventricular blocking.

The common and convenient division into congenital and acquired has, in part, a more substantial anatomical basis.

On this question of the congenital form the results of a study of the spinal absorbents, given in another article, have an important bearing. But it must remain for a closer examination of such cases from this new point of view to show more exactly what the relation is.

CONGENITAL HYDROCEPHALUS.

While it is not proposed here to take up this class, a word may be said regarding it in passing. Of this form we have but a poor knowledge. There is a supposition that it depends on other conditions or causes than the acquired form. Yet the same principles must be involved, at least so far as the immediate cause of the retention. In the elaborate description of Hans Virchow ("Ein Fall von angeborenem Hydrocephalus Internus," etc., Leipzig, 1887) there is evidence that in his case the fluid was not pent up in the ventricles, but had connection with the general subarachnoid space. It was due to a chronic lepto-meningitis which evidently had sealed up the ultimate absorbents.

Some other congenital cases are included in lists given below.

ACQUIRED HYDROCEPHALUS.

Various explanations according to the case have been offered to account for the increase of fluid. The most tenable are,—

a. Closure of the canal from the ventricles, particularly at Magendie's foramen,—retention of fluid.

b. Interference with the venous discharge, in particular of Galen's vein,—over-production of fluid.

c. Inflammation or other irritation of the choroidal villi *

---

* Kindfleisch ("Pathol. Anat.") is credited as one of the first to insist on the rôle of lesions of the choroid plexus in the production of cœlian dropsy.

in the ventricles (ependymitis, hyperplasia of the choroid plexus, meningitis serosa, tubercular meningitis, etc.),—also increased production.

These causes of themselves do not offer an explanation of the retention, and more careful examination at autopsies will somewhat reduce the apparent frequency of such cases. Even in tubercular meningitis it not rarely transpires that there is ample obstruction from specially situated tubercular or inflammatory material to explain the accumulation.

d. The stretching form of Huguenin, occurring only in the young (a kind of passive or relative retention). This is supposed to be due to abnormally diminished resistance of the cranial walls from malnutrition and imperfect development. Here rickets and hereditary syphilis play the chief rôle. Or it is attributed to the head strain of coughing (pertussis, chronic bronchitis, etc.). On the balloon-valve principle, and in view of the fact that the spinal absorbents are shut off soon after birth, this is conceivable. The efforts of coughing fill up the brain and so press it against the cranial absorbents as to impede their efficient action.

But this theory is opposed by the large experience of Heubner (see his article in Eulenberg's "Cyclopædie").

e. This classification, however, does not offer from the mechanical stand-point a satisfactory explanation except in part.

To these forms we must logically add another, due to obstruction of the ultimate absorbents from the subarachnoid space, whatever the nature of these absorbents, or however they act (*v. supra*, special article). The occurrence of suspended material in some cases, that must be carried along, suggests one way by which the eventual outlets may be stopped up. The local inflammation of a meningitis constitutes another. The balloon-valve principle represents a third. This last could not be accorded much importance so long as not only cranial but also spinal absorbents were supposed to exist. But it has already been shown that there are no spinal efferents after the first weeks of infancy. Hence any distention of, or increase of pressure from the side of, the brain proper must materially interfere with the usefulness of the remaining—*i.e.*, cranial—outlets.

Either we must acknowledge such a form, or else, what is equivalent to it, a relative insufficiency of the absorbents when extra demands are placed on them. As yet we do not know with any exactness the normal rate of production of the cerebro-spinal fluid, and still less the quantitative ability of the absorbents to carry it off. Since, however, the spinal absorbents become obsolete soon after birth, while as yet the cranial absorbents (*in specie* the Pacchionian villi) have not acquired the scope of adult and later life, it is clear that in the early period (infancy and childhood) the ultimate absorbents are very much restricted and *their quantitative ability may far more readily show a relative insufficiency.* Herein may be one long-sought reason for the greater frequency of hydrocephalus in early life.*

---

* The matter of hydrocephalus in childhood, aside from the congenital form, is a somewhat different one from that in adults. Its greater frequency is due to several causes,—

1st. The scant absorbents, peculiar to this period, as just pointed out.

2d. The narrowness of the passages. This allows of their occlusion, whether by inflammatory process, pressure, or direct plugging, much more readily than in adults.

3d. To a slight extent it may be due to the yielding nature of the cranium at that age. This has long figured as a favorite cause, but it bears rather on the volume than the frequency of the effusion.

This form (*e*) includes *c*, and must play an important part in *b*, and even the uncertain *d*. If this plan were strictly carried out, we should put all cases of internal hydrocephalus, congenital as well as acquired, under two chief divisions, corresponding to *a* (central retention) and *e* (arachnoidal retention),—all other types then becoming subforms, according to their etiology. While this is, without doubt, a correct classification, and a necessary one from the mechanical stand-point, sufficient facts for a complete study of form *e* are wanting.

The thorough establishing of certain provisional forms, as *a* and *b*, is an almost necessary preliminary to the general acceptance of such a division as that just indicated. The accumulated evidence showing the reality of these two forms amounts to a demonstration. They include all cases due to direct interference with the outflow from the ventricles of either *A*, the cerebro-spinal fluid, or *B*, the blood in the veins. The channels for such discharge will now be briefly described.

VENTRICULAR EFFERENTS.

A. FOR THE CEREBRO-SPINAL FLUID.

This is produced by the choroid plexuses in the ventricles. That from the paracœles is augmented from the plexuses in the diacœle and metacœle on the way out.

4th. The relatively larger size of the emanating vein of Galen, as compared with that in adults (from the writer's observations probable), suggests a more important rôle for the ventricular circulation in childhood. There is likewise, according to Trolard, more cerebro-spinal fluid, comparatively, than in the adult up to the senile conditions. But it is possible that his observation is explained by the limitation of absorbents.

5th. The provoking causes, such as tubercular meningitis, are more frequent in the early years of life.

1. The only normal exit from the lateral ventricles is per foramen of Munro, third ventricle, aqueduct of Sylvius, and fourth ventricle. From this last to the general subarachnoid space there are the metapore (foramen of Magendie) and the lesser aperturæ laterales (*a. l. ventriculi quarti* of Key and Retzius, foramina Luschkæ).

Other described exits from the ventricles are evidently artefacts.

The experimental injections of Key and Retzius in Sweden, corroborated by Marc Sée in France and by Fischer and Waldeyer in Germany, have furnished the anatomical proof that this view, previously indicated by Magendie and worked out by Hilton from pathological cases, is correct.

The foramen of Magendie is described as an opening through the tela choroidea inferior. Magendie gave it an average breadth of two to three lines. Luschka says it is often six lines long and four broad. According to Wilder (*Jrnl. Nev. and Mnt. Dis.*, 1886, p. 207), "The mesal foramen of Magendie is approximately rhomboidal in outline, about five millimetres wide and eight to ten millimetres long." Frequently small vessels and fibres cross this opening from oblongata to cerebellum.

Renault, Luschka (1855), and also Key and Retzius found that in the horse, and perhaps in some other animals, this posterior aperture is normally absent, the laterals, however, being so much the larger.

Key and Retzius say the aperturæ laterales empty into the cisterna magna cerebello-medullaris, and that they are so filled up by the villi of the plexus choroideus lateralis as to favor the exit of fluid but impede the reverse.

Through the upper part of this aperture on each side,

beside the median line of the anterior two-thirds of the infravermis, runs, according to Luschka, the middle portion of this plexus, its course showing the necessary existence of an opening.

That the ventricular fluid flows through the aqueduct of Sylvius into the fourth ventricle, and then out through the lateral apertures as well as the metapore, was practically shown by the autopsy recorded on p. 129, Case I. Such cases of hemorrhage, not very rare in any pathologist's experience, show that this channel is the natural outlet. Of course, it is also not rare at autopsy to find that an hemorrhagic effusion has travelled along this route, but in just the opposite direction.

2. Possibly also by certain lymphatics. Ependymal stomata have been described. It has even been assumed that the choroidal villi both secrete and absorb fluid. Such efferents are, however, uncertain, and, in this connection, of scant importance.

"The lymphatics of the choroid plexus in the paracœles unite (Arnold) to form one trunk, following Galen's vein. In the ependyma lymphatic net-works have occasionally been observed" (from author's article in Buck's "Reference Hand-Book"). Whether such exist or then really absorb ventricular fluid is not very material, since, of themselves, they are unable to head off an hydrocephalus when the aqueduct-path is once closed. Hence they are, at most, but accessory exits. It is a question of the natural outlets for the fluid. If it be reabsorbed locally, then it does not go to the general stock of cephalo-rachidian liquor, and apparently fails of its main purpose. Quincke's experiments failed to show such absorption, but pointed to the path out as above described.

The matter of the ultimate absorption of the fluid from the subarachnoid space is considered in a special article.

B. For the Blood.

This is conducted off by the vein of Galen and its affluents, discharging through the sinus rectus. Hence the anastomotic connections of this vessel and its branches acquire a considerable importance. It receives several accessions from the cortex, each of which has connections sufficient to provide collateral discharge in case of its individual occlusion. Or these together might serve as substitute efferents for the main trunk of Galen. These cortical branches otherwise play no part in hydrocephalus. The main question hinges on the real ventricular vessels, the two venæ intimæ (velars), with their sources in the cœlian walls, and the venæ choroideæ.

1. The cortical branches of Galen's vein are the basilar, the supercerebellar, the suboccipital, and the (azygos) callosal.

In only one-half the cases in man, as was shown by the writer, does the basilar (the largest external branch) come up around the resp. crus cerebri to empty into the corresponding vena intima or more directly into the vena Galeni, Only in such can it adapt itself as a collateral and serve to convey blood in the opposite direction (*i.e.*, out of the ventricle).

The suboccipital, supercerebellar, and callosal veins, emptying at about the same point as the basilar, might also be available as anastomoses. At best this can only occur when the obstruction is strictly limited to the sinus rectus or the adjacent portion of the short trunk of Galen's vein. If the obstruction extends peripherally beyond the specified venous channel, then, of course, these cortical connections cannot act as collaterals.

But in one-half the cases in man the basilar vein has merely a nominal connection with the ventricular vessels, and then, of course, is not available. This statement refers, however, to the individual sides, and, as in a given subject this vessel frequently takes the upper course on one side while its partner of the opposite side remains basal, it follows that only in the minority of cases is this alternative outlet for the azygous vena Galeni altogether wanting. In this latter type blockage of Galen's vein or the straight sinus becomes, from an anatomical stand-point, a more serious affair, though the other collaterals mentioned might still suffice.

2. Velars,—the ventricular veins in the strict sense.

Two particular lines for collateral discharge, in case of blockage of one or both these veins, must be considered.

First. The one is by means of the subcornual vein, first specially described by the writer. This is a considerable vessel that arises in the walls of the inferior horn, connects freely with the branches of the choroidal vein in the fringe of plexus that runs down the infracornu (much as the anterior and middle choroid arteries inosculate), and, after passing out at the extreme lateral tip of Bichat's fissure, empties into the basilar vein. It was possibly by this round-about and not altogether certain inosculation that compensation was established in Wenzel's case (*v. infra*, p. 87). As a general thing, however, it must be an impractical substitute.

Second. Per trans-albal connections with cortical veins.

I have elsewhere sought to show that the velar branches,

from the substance of the hemispheres, were terminal vessels. But Hédon, a later French investigator, claims that these veins do have more or less connection, through their fine ramifications in the brain-substance, with those discharging at the brain-surface. Even, however, granting such connections,—and I have seen, as well as drawn, the particular veinlets for which he makes the claim,—they are very small, traverse the hemispheres for a long distance, and, as experience amply shows, are inadequate for collateral purposes.

Two facts become apparent after any careful consideration of the evidence in normal and pathological cases. First, that in practice it is rare to find a case with compression, or other obstruction to the current in the straight sinus or Galen's vein, in which there is not also more or less interference with these possible collaterals. Second, that any considerable disturbance of the customary venous exit from the cœles induces a marked increase in the production of the fluid, anastomoses or no anastomoses. Perhaps it also changes unfavorably the character of the fluid produced.

There is another lesser vein, but as important in its smaller field,—the "floccular vein," first described by the writer.* There is one on each side. It derives a large branch from the plexus in the lateral recess of the fourth ventricle. This "choroid plexus emerges from the lateral recess near the flocculus, between the seventh and eighth nerves anteriorly, and the glosso-pharyngeal posteriorly" (Sutton). It may join with the basilar when this empties at the base.

---

* "Veins of the Brain," pp. 36, 37.

THE EFFECT OF OBSTRUCTION OF THESE EFFERENT PASSAGES.

A'. AT VARIOUS POINTS IN THE PATH OF THE VENTRICU-
LAR (CEREBRO-SPINAL) FLUID.

In cases of tumor in any of the ventricles it is often difficult to make out, especially after removal of the brain, how much blockage there may have been to either class of efferents ; and hence impossible to say just what the bearing of the case may be on the matter here in question. Some cases involving the paracœles will be given later under venous obstruction.

The points at issue can best be determined by a study of obstruction at the orifices or small parts of the passage. No attempt will be made to give an exhaustive collection of published cases, but enough from accessible sources to illustrate.

1. In troubles in the lateral ventricles, associated with a collection of fluid, the exact relation of the two often cannot be made out. Still, it is easy to see that neoplasms, adhesions, etc., may impede either the fluid or venous discharge, and so in principle conform to what will be shown farther along.

It is known, since Virchow's description, that obstruction of a posterior horn causes a dilatation of the part cut off. And Bland Sutton has described (*Brain*, October, 1886) similar cystic formations from obstructions in the lateral recesses of the fourth ventricle. In the latter location we must assume a double or complete closing-in to explain a cyst, unless regarded as part of the whole ventricle. In any of these partial forms a bit of choroid plexus must be included that fluid can accumulate therefrom.

2. At the Foramen of Munro.

As it is by this passage that the laterals connect with the third ventricle, it is clear that its closure suffices to cut off the outlet from one or both the laterals, and so dam back their discharge.

Cases of sacculated fluid representing a part of one ventricle have just been referred to. When, however, the effusion fills the whole of one lateral and is limited to that, there is a closure on the affected side of the opening into the third ventricle. Or, as Gowers in more general terms says, when "confined to one or both lateral ventricles, there is some obstruction at the foramen of Munro."

1'. In Reynolds's "System of Medicine" a case is given from Vrolik ("Traité sur l'Hydrocephalie interne," Amsterdam, 1839) "of a young man who died from chronic hydrocephalus at the age of twenty, and in whom a false membrane had occluded the foramen of Munro."

2'. Broxholm, *Lancet*, 1853, ii. p. 349. Woman of twenty-seven years. No premonitory symptoms except a headache for twelve hours. "On removing the skull-cap about a pint of serum escaped, and the vessels appeared very much congested; the sinuses were completely engorged. On slitting down the brain and opening the lateral ventricles, they were found much distended with fluid, and between the layers of the septum lucidum (the fifth ventricle) a hydatid cyst, the size of a small marble, was detected floating in fluid." While this may not have been a direct closure of Munro's foramen, it evidently had that effect.

3'. Förster (*Würzburger Med. Ztschr.*, 1864, p. 39, quoted by Edes, *Med. News*, 1888, i. p. 61, Case I.): "Ventricles found moderately enlarged, filled with clear water, and a growth in the median line of the choroid plexus, which had evidently caused the hydrocephalus. The growth was in the middle ventricle, directly at and partly in the much-enlarged foramen of Munro."

4'. Edés's own case (*ibid.*, p. 62) : "In the lateral ventricles were six ounces of clear serum. In the choroid plexus and directly in the foramen of Munro was a soft grayish, rounded tumor."

5'. W. W. Keen, *Med. News*, September 20, 1890, p. 277, Case III. : "This was a case of tubercular meningitis, with unilateral acute internal hydrocephalus of the left ventricle. The foramen of Munro, as determined at the autopsy, was closed. This closure was attended by unilateral distention, and produced right hemiplegia."

6'. Baskett, *Brit. Med. Jrnl.*, 1894, i. p. 63, relates a case of tapping for relief of a congenital hydrocephalus. After this there was a gradual but unilateral accumulation, due to plugging at foramen of Munro.

3. Third Ventricle.

Growths here rarely obstruct the passage for fluid without also involving the veins above, or possibly irritating the choroidal fringes and so limiting their significance. Yet there are sufficient cases for illustration.

1'. Coindet, quoted by Lallemand (p. 184 of the German edition of his work on the brain, Leipzig, 1825). Girl of seven months. In the right lateral was about half a pound of chocolate-colored mixture of blood and brain-substance. The left ventricle contained nearly twelve ounces of clear serous fluid. No trace of the third ventricle ("der dritte Ventrikel war gar nicht mehr vorhanden").

2'. H. Wallmann, *Virch. Arch.*, 1858, Bd. xiv. p. 385. Man of fifty-two years. Colloid cyst of third ventricle connected with the plexus choroideus medius and posterior commissure. It measured three and one-fifth centimetres in length by one and three-fifths centimetres in breadth and thickness. It was situated a little posteriorly in the third ventricle, and this cœle was formed to the outlines of the tumor. Great internal hydrocephalus. As, however, the fornix was pressed upward, there may have been some vein-interference.

3'. Woodbury, *Am. Jrnl. Med. Sc.*, July, 1878 : "Tumor, size of a walnut, found in the ventricle, moulded to the interior." "A caudate prolongation completely blocked the iter." Fourth, [?] and to a less extent lateral ventricles enormously distended.

4'. Bristowe, *Brain*, 1884, pp. 182–184, Case III. : "Much distention of lateral ventricles with clear fluid. The third ventricle was occupied by an irregularly globular tubercular mass, one and one-half inches in diameter, which partly involved both optic thalami." Ended with tubercular meningitis.

5'. In Dana's case (*Jrnl. Nrv. and Mnt. Dis.*, 1892, p. 217) "there was no great excess of fluid in the ventricles."

4. Aqueduct of Sylvius.

A narrow, easily occluded passage.* It is quite as prob-

---

* Boenninghaus has recently (" Die Meningitis serosa," Wiesbaden, 1897) described what he calls active closure of the ventricular outlet at this passage, —in contrast to what he calls passive closure by actual sealing up at any point along the ventricular outlet,—and attributes to this many cases of collection in lateral and third ventricles to the exclusion of the fourth. He conceives that first a secretion of fluid occurs faster than the aqueduct can carry it off. This secondarily so drags on the aqueduct as to close it. Of course, in such a case, after removal of the brain nothing remains to show the manner of blocking. He also applies a similar scheme to the outlets from the fourth ventricle. It, however, can hardly be claimed that there is any real evidence in favor of such a theory.

able that cerebellar tumors produce an aggregation of fluid in the paracœles by pressure on this fine exit, as on the vein of Galen. More limited and unmistakable obstruction of this duct is, however, occasionally recorded.

1'. Hilton, "On Rest and Pain," gives the post-mortem of a girl of seven months, who had been hydrocephalic since four months old. "The lateral ventricles were distended, and contained four ounces of fluid." "The iter e tertio ad quartem ventriculum was dilated nearly as far as the entrance into the fourth ventricle, where it was closed by old and firm adhesion. This occlusion necessarily preserved the fourth ventricle from dilatation, and it was accordingly natural in form."

2'. Bristowe, *Brain*, 1884, p. 188, Case V. Man of seventeen years. Lateral ventricles largely and uniformly dilated. These communicated freely with the large and distended third ventricle. The commencement of the iter was quite blocked by a translucent septum, looking like a portion of the ependyma. The fourth ventricle was distended with fluid and formed a cyst isolated from all the other cœles. Oblongata and first six inches of cord much enlarged, but quite independently of the fourth ventricle.

3'. A case of Taylor's is quoted by Goodhart, of London (*Arch. of Pediatrics*, 1888, p. 39), in which there was a congenital hydrocephalus, and where at the autopsy the Sylvian aqueduct was found obliterated.

4'. Nothnagel (*Wien. Med. Blätter*, 1888, No. 6, *v. Centbl. f. Med. Wissc.*, 1888, p. 578). Man of seventeen years. Besides usual symptoms of brain-pressure there was a repeated outflow of cerebro-spinal fluid from right nostril and even eye. A firm, hazel-nut-sized tumor of the corpora quadrigemina was found pressing down on the aqueduct of

Sylvius, and in the posterior portion completely closing it. The ventricles, except the fourth, were greatly dilated and filled with fluid.

5'. Chaffey, *Brit. Med. Jrnl.*, 1891, ii. p. 224. Tapping of lateral ventricles. Death. The "dilatation was doubtless mainly induced by a caseous deposit at the summit of the transverse fissure, which pressed upon and constricted the iter." Some recent tubercles in the Sylvian fissure also.

6'. Jos. Collins, *Am. Jrnl. Med. Sc.*, October, 1895, pp. 420–425. Youth of eighteen years. Lateral ventricles found greatly distended (eight to ten ounces escaped), and practically continuous with third. The fourth ventricle contained no fluid. (At another point he speaks of "the distention of the fourth ventricle," but this is evidently a mistake). "Grayish translucent mass filling the aqueduct of Sylvius and projecting backward like a tongue." It extended just about the full length of the iter.

7'. In marked contrast to the above is the unique case of Quincke (Volkmann's "Sammlung," N. F., No. 67, 1893, pp. 687, 688), where the aqueduct was congenitally closed (boy of about six months), but the third ventricle in some way communicated with the subarachnoid space. The lateral ventricles were much dilated.

Tumors of the quadrigeminal region are rarely in point, as they so easily compress both the iter and Galen's vein. Typical here are tumors of the pineal gland. A review of the cases of Birch-Hirschfeld, Fontoppidian, Reinhold, Schulz, and Zenner fully justifies the statement of the latter (*Alienist and Neurologist*, 1892, p. 470), based on his own and nine previous cases. "All these were much alike. Usually the tumor was described as the size of a walnut, and as pressing on neighboring organs, especially the corpora quadrigemina. A special feature was pressure on the vena Galeni, or aqueduct of Sylvius, which caused internal hydrocephalus." In these cases the fourth ventricle is, of course, not included in the hydrocephalus.

5. The Fourth Ventricle.

This is the next stage caudad in the path of the fluid. About the only evidence available to show what closure of this cavity will do is furnished by cases of local neoplasm. Such growths may not suffice to cut off the way. Evidently this was the condition in Schmidt's case (*Jrnl. Nerv. and Mnt. Dis.*, 1882), where there were two growths, one on each side, and, in the absence of further information, very likely also in that of Edes (*Boston M. and S. J.*, 1896, ii. p. 410).

Audry, in his article on tumors of the choroid plexus (*Rev. de Médc.*, Nov., 1886), recognizes the fact that they are usually complicated by hydrocephalus due to vein or fluid obstruction. In seven of his series of collected cases it is specifically stated that there was ventricular accumulation with tumor of the metepicœle,—viz., in the cases of (1') Robin, 1858 ; (2') Levrat-Perroton, 1859 ; (3') Zenker, 1871 ; (4') Garrod, 1873 ; (5') Recklinghausen, 1874 ; (6') Spillmann, 1882; and (7') Douty, 1885.

8'. Ogle, *Trans. Path. Soc.*, London, 1856, vol. vii. Boy of eight years. Acute hydrocephalus from exposure to sun three years previously. Tough membrane surrounding a cyst of the whole fourth ventricle ; lateral ventricles very large, containing not less than a pint.

9'. Charles Kelly, *ibid.*, 1873, vol. xxiv. Boy of eleven years. A papilloma was found, very much distending the ventricle. " The lateral ventricles were full of clear serous fluid."

10'. Another specially good case is given by Anton ("Zur Anatomie des Hydrocephalus und des Hirndruckes," *Wien. Med. Jahrb.*, 1888, quoted by G. Levi, *Königsberg Dissertation*, 1896). Man of twenty years, who had suffered six years from symptoms of brain-pressure. An echinococcus with surrounding thickened tissue completely closed the fourth ventricle.

11'. Quincke, "Ueber Meningitis serosa," Leipzig, 1893, p. 684. Male of twenty-one years. Duration of special symptoms about six months. Marked hydrocephalic distention of lateral and third ventricles. Aqueduct of Sylvius greatly dilated. Fourth ventricle filled with a soft glioma.

12'. *Ibid.*, p. 685. Brief reference to another case of hydrocephalus due to a cyst in the fourth ventricle, originating from the cerebellum.

13'. F. Pick, *Ztschr. f. Heilkunde*, Bd. xiii. (*v. Neurlgc. Centbl.*, 1893, p. 278). Man of thirty-seven years, who had presented symptoms of brain-tumor. Autopsy showed a complete closure of the fourth ventricle by a cicatricial formation in front of the alæ cinerea. This involved the ependyma of the fovea rhomboidalis, the anterior extremity of the infravermis, and the plexus choroideus. It had produced a high degree of hydrocephalus. Etiology uncertain.

14'. Bruns, reported in *Neurlgc. Centbl.*, 1895, p. 521. Sarcoma, size of a medium apple, in fourth ventricle of a boy of five years. Symptoms began in his second year. Enormous hydrocephalus.

15'. Kretz, "Tod durch Hydrocephalus nach intermeningealer Blutung aus einem Aneurysma der Arteria carotis interna," *Wiener klin. Wochr.*, 1895, No. 33 (*v. Neurlgc. Centbl.*, 1896, p. 655.) Man of thirty-nine years. "The cavity of the fourth ventricle was closed by adhesion of the tela choroidea to the fovea rhomboidalis. Chronic hydrocephalus." The adhesions were attributed to a heavy intermeningeal hemorrhage from the aneurism, corresponding to a severe apoplectic attack eight months antemortem.

6. The observation of a closure of the cerebro-spinal foramen (the foramen Magendie of Luschka, Hilton's canal, Apertura inferior ventriculi quarti of Key and Retzius, Wilder's metapore) in cases of hydrocephalus has been repeatedly corroborated, although not to the extent of finding this particular opening obstructed in nearly every case, as was Hilton's experience.

1', 2', and 3'. According to Key and Retzius (1875, p. 117), Magendie * found this communication closed twice in elderly individuals. There was an abnormal quantity of fluid in the ventricles in each case. Both subjects were insane.

And Magendie cited another case from Martin Saint-Ange. This occurred in a child of eight years. There had been severe cerebral symptoms. The ventricles were filled with much serum, and the foramen of Magendie was closed by a pretty firm opaque membrane.

4' and 5'. Hilton, in his work on "Rest and Pain," published two cases more in detail, the first dating from 1844.

6' and 7'. Hanot and Joffroy, *Gaz. Méd.*, 1873 (*v.* Wernicke). Opacity and thickening of pia. Posteriorly the adhesions were so strong that the cerebellum was firmly attached to the oblongata. Dilatation of the ventricles.

---

* Presumably published in his "Recherches sur le liquide céphalo-rachidien," Paris, 1842, although I have not been able to see the original.

In a second case of theirs, a man of seventeen years made a relative recovery from meningitis, then suddenly died. The cerebellum was so closely adherent to the bulbus that the pia had to be cut through with scissors. Here also the fourth ventricle was dilated.

8' to 23'. At the London Pathl. Soc. (meeting of February 21, 1882; abstract in *Med. Ti. and Gaz.* of March 4) several cases were reported, by Drs Baxter (one), Mackenzie (three), and Lees (a dozen more).

24'. Bunce, *Edinburgh Med. Jrnl.*, March, 1887, p. 838. Girl. Simple meningitis. Apparent recovery. Convulsions and death. "On looking at the under surface of the cerebellum and medulla the fibrous thickening of the membrane had formed an adhesion between the two sides of the latter and amygdala, which were also closely united." "Lateral ventricles were found considerably distended. The foramen of Munro was dilated to have a diameter of about half an inch." "The third ventricle was also dilated, as was the fourth. The pineal gland was normal, and the two veins of Galen not at all obstructed. It was probable that the increase of fluid was due to the blocking up of the lymphatic outlet at the foramen of Magendie, caused by the gluing of the cerebellum to the sides of the medulla."

25'. F. Plehn (*Kiel Dissertation*, 1887) gives the case of a student of twenty-three years, who had suffered much from cephalalgia since an accident in his tenth year. Sudden death under signs of suffocation. Great distention of lateral, third, and fourth ventricles by fluid. Aqueduct permeable. Foramen of Magendie obliterated. Pia in post-cerebellar region whitish, opaque, and thickened.

26'. In a case from Dr. Habershon's service at Guy's

Hospital in 1871 (No. 6 of Fagge's "System of Medicine," 1888, i. p. 661) Magendie's opening was found closed.

27'. Lawson, of Hull (*Brit. Med. Jrnl.*, 1893, i. p. 1322). One case of evident closure of foramen of Magendie in connection with hydrocephalus.

28' and 29'. Two cases of hydrocephalus—one in a boy of thirteen and a half years, and the other in a girl of four years, associated with complete àbsence of communication between the fourth ventricle and the subarachnoid space— have recently been described by O'Carroll (*Trans. Irish Acad. Mcdc.*, 1894). Here it is specifically noted that the lateral exits were also closed.

30'. Neurath, *Aerztl. Central-Anzg.*, 1895, Wien, vii. p. 521. Boy of eleven years. Hydrocephalus began six years before, presumably from a scarlatinal leptomeningitis. Brain-ventricles were greatly distended, and contained about half a litre of clear fluid. The third ventricle bulged downward. Aqueductus Sylvii distended to size of a crow's quill. The fourth ventricle was cystically enlarged to size of a nut. The foramen of Magendie was closed ; the arachnoidea and pia were here closely grown together and somewhat opaque. No dilatation of central canal of cord.

31'. Key and Retzius (1875, p. 117) give a case where they found a thin film, as a direct continuation of the tela choroidea inferior, closing this opening. And yet there was no abnormal effusion in the ventricles. They specify that it was certainly not of inflammatory or neoplastic origin, but perhaps embryonic. On page 122, however, they state that the lateral apertures from the fourth ventricle were in this case open.

The argument of most writers that, because every case of hydrocephalus is not due to obstruction at just this point, such a cause is very doubtful, simply ignores the fact that this particular seat of obstruction does not hold for all cases.   It is time to recognize its full and complete validity wherever found.   That upon the very principle upon which obstruction at this point acts, there are plenty of cases where the particular location is at some other point, is an integral part of the explanation.   The main matter in this theory is further not affected by any question as to whether the occlusion be limited strictly to the foramen of Magendie or whether, together with this, the other small adjacent communications (aperturæ laterales, more or less filled by choroid plexus) be also closed.   In O'Carroll's two cases the latter condition was found ; the same holds for Pick's case, and in the others cited there is fair reason to conclude that it also existed.

While, as stated, this explanation applies, of course, only to cases in which such obstruction is present, it harmonizes perfectly with that for the previous cases of interference higher up, and goes far towards establishing a general theory of obstructive hydrocephalus.

The case of Key and Retzius, where with closure of the foramen of Magendie the lateral apertures were open and no fluid stasis occurred, and the later ones of O'Carroll, where all these apertures were closed and the stasis did occur, serve to definitely round out the picture and complete the final proof.   If further clinching is necessary, it is afforded by the successful results of English operators, to which fuller reference will be made under treatment.   In following out this view to its practical application by re-opening the metapore, they have achieved a fair share of cures.

A natural query might be, What becomes of the continual flow of ventricular fluid if all outlets are shut off?

In the first place, it is possible that a minimal quantity may pass outward through the surrounding tissue, or by way of the uncertain cœlian lymphatics described as accompanying Galen's vein. Another portion is stored up in the increasing hydrocephalus. For the most part, however, the counter-pressure must greatly retard the production of the fluid. If a little rise in venous pressure serves to materially increase the production, then, *per contra*, a resisting pressure must very materially check it.

B'. FROM OBSTRUCTION TO THE VENOUS DISCHARGE.

As an exclusive cause this is infrequent and less effective than interference with the fluid-discharge. The principle plays its chief part in those numerous cases where there is partial obstruction to both the venous and fluid exits from the cœles.

Our first knowledge of the fact that internal hydrocephalus may be due to obstruction of the vein of Galen is credited to Whytt ("Observations on the Dropsy in the Brain, by Robert Whytt, M.D.," Edinburgh, 1768). All he says is, in speaking "Of the Causes of a Dropsy in the Ventricles of the Brain," as cause 3 : "A scirrhous tumor of the glandula pituitaria, or in any part contiguous to the ventricles of the brain, by compressing the neighboring trunks of the absorbent veins will prevent the due absorption of that fluid which the small arteries constantly exhale, and occasion a dropsy in the brain, in like manner as a scirrhous liver, spleen, or pancreas are often the cause of an ascites. As a proof of this we may observe that M. Petit often found the glandula pituitaria scirrhous in those who died of a dropsy of the ventricles of the brain.

"In one case I met with a hard tumor within the right

thalamus nervorum opticorum.   It was almost as large as a small hen's egg, of a yellowish color within, and of a firm consistence."

There is some ground to question Whytt's claim to recognition here.   He certainly does not suggest that interference with this vein increases the output of fluid, but only that it interferes with a supposed venous absorption. Later work has shown that the veins are not the absorbents of the fluid.   Hence, in any strict sense, much of the credit belongs to later men, especially as regards any correct interpretation of facts.

In hunting for the immediate cause of any obscure case of hydrocephalus the venous outlets from the cœles should be subjected to careful scrutiny.

The peculiar course of Galen's vein, as observed by Braune and described by the writer,* exposes it greatly to compression.   Especially will any encroachment of the post-cranial fossa exert pressure in the direction of least resistance,—i.e., towards the incisura tentorii.   This compresses the vein laterally against the splenium, and hence in the most effective manner.

Another weak spot here is the slit through the tentorium, by which this vein discharges into the beginning of the straight sinus.   Pressure upward on the middle of the tentorium, or even against the falx in front of the opening, must tend to draw the slit tighter, and so shut off the outflow.

---

* Some previous illustrations had pictured, more or less correctly, the angle at which this vein enters the straight sinus.   For example, it is fairly well shown in the work of Key and Retzius (Erste Hälfte, 1875, Taf. vii. Fig. 1). But no notice had ever been taken of it, or of the vein's long curve around the splenium.

1. Walman, *Virch. Arch.*, 1858, Bd. xiv. p. 385. An old soldier. The ventricles were found dilated. Under the fornix was an oval tumor the size of a nut. It was adherent by its posterior border to the median choroid plexus, and was also adherent to the posterior commissure. (Possibly this may have also pressed on the commencement of the iter.) Lipoma size of a bean in right lateral plexus.

2. David Newman, *Glasgow Med. Jrnl.*, September, 1882, p. 163, Case II. Ventricular hydrocephalus due to thrombosis of Galen's vein. Man, aged fifty-five years. "Until three months before death the patient enjoyed perfect health. Symptoms began with vertigo, lassitude, disturbed sleep at night, and drowsiness during the day ; but patient was sufficiently well to follow his occupation until six days prior to death, when he suddenly became comatose, and showed evidence of left hemiplegia, and afterwards of general muscular paralysis. There were no convulsions or spasmodic movements, but slight convergent strabismus was noticed with dilatation of pupils. Sphincters unaffected. Slight recovery of mental powers two days before death, succeeded by sudden relapse.

"*Post-mortem Inspection.*—External appearance presents nothing remarkable. *Head.*—The bones of the head are firmly united, and there is no evident increase in size, nor are the eyeballs protruded. The *dura mater* is slightly thickened and unusually tense. The superior longitudinal sinus is empty. The Pacchionian bodies are enlarged and project slightly into the cavity of the sinus. There are no morbid changes, fatty, atheromatous, or aneurismal, in the vessels at the base of the brain, except, perhaps, a suspicious yellow spot in the artery of the fissure of Sylvius on the left side. The cerebral convolutions are flattened, soft, and œdematous, but there is no fluid collected in the arachnoid. The lateral ventricles are considerably dilated by an accumulation of about four and a half ounces of clear, straw-colored fluid in each of them. The structures forming the floor of the lateral ventricles are soft, flattened, and œdematous ; the choroid plexus is unusually vascular, and contains a few small cysts, and, tracing the vessels of the plexus backward, a small, whitish, moderately firm, and adherent clot is found in the vein of Galen, close to its union with the inferior longitudinal and straight sinuses ; the thrombosis does not pass beyond the opening of Galen's vein ; and it may be observed, further, that in none of the other vessels or sinuses are any clots seen. Spinal cord normal."

(Other organs of the body showed unimportant or no changes.)

"*Chemical and Microscopic Examination of Fluid from Ventricles of Brain.*—Fluid of a straw color, sp. gr. 1007, contains .501 per cent. of solid matter, and on microscopic examination of the sediment a few leucocytes and one or two crystals of cholesterine and margarine are seen.

"ANALYSIS OF FLUID.

Water	994.99
Solids :	
Albuminous matter	.91
Fatty	.26
Alcoholic extract	.41
Other organic matter (mostly alcapton) . .	.60
Inorganic salts	2.83
	5.01
	1000.00"

P. 165. In this "case the patient was old, the progress of the disease rapid, and there was no enlargement of the head ; and, beyond thrombosis of Galen's vein, and as a consequence the accumulation of fluid in the ventricles, with flattening of the convolutions, there were no morbid changes discovered in the brain."

"The obstruction to the venous flow from the choroid plexus, etc., was complete, and evidently sudden."

P. 167. "In all the cases we have found recorded, the thrombi have passed beyond Galen's vein into the straight, lateral, or longitudinal sinuses, so that the case above described seems to be quite unique."

The moderate degree of distention in this case may have been due to the unyielding cranium, or in part, at least, to that cause.

3. J. Stedman (*Bost. M. and S. J.*, August 9, 1883, and 1891, vol. i. pp. 82, 83, Case IV.). "Lateral ventricles distended at least a third larger than usual, and filled with clear, watery fluid." "A gray, gelatinous tumor, the size of a filbert, was found upon the velum interpositum, in the median line, behind the fifth ventricle, in the region of the anterior commissure, on a level with the junction of the corpora striata and optic thalami." A cystic tumor easily removed from its surroundings. "The structure and seat of the tumor suggested its origin from the choroid plexus ; its position upon the venæ Galeni (velars ?) explained satisfactorily the dropsy of the ventricles."

4. K. Wenzel, "Ein Fall von Hydrocephalus internus chronicus acquisitus." Bonn, 1886.

It has been claimed that in this case Magendie's foramen was closed, but a careful reading of the original fails to find any proof that such was the fact.

The patient was a girl, three and one-third years old at death ; bottle-fed as infant ; convulsions at ten weeks and beginning hydrocephalus three months later,—due, as he concludes, to a leptomeningitis infantum. Puncture of ventricle was first practised three and a half months before death. This yielded a non-inflammatory fluid, of which a detailed analysis is given. A second puncture was also made.

At the autopsy, one to one and a half litres of fluid came from the enormously dilated lateral ventricles. "The pia at the base, especially from chiasm to pons, was much thickened, firm, and opaque;" but there were no tubercles.

"Very numerous and noticeable small veins run from the large ganglia [central] up and outward on the lateral wall of the paracœles. . . . The plexus choroideus was of a lively red, rolled almost together, and quite granular and firm. It doubled around, following the fimbria fornicis from the infracornu, shrunk up noticeably opposite the thalamus, and, turning towards the quadrigemina, vanished without continuing out in a median portion. From this extremity of the plexus, veins pass outward which correspond in part to the stria terminalis ; and it appears that blood can be forced from the end of the plexus into these above-described veins running up and outward. Nothing is to be seen of a median choroid plexus. Third ventricle very wide ; anterior and posterior commissures intact. . . . The floor of the fourth ventricle is formed of a translucent, very compact, and resisting membrane. . . . Fourth ventricle showed no abnormity."

"From the front upper extremity of the cerebellar supravermis to the splenium corporis callosi stretched a firm fibrous membrane, completely closing up the great brainfissure. . . . There was a compact, stout adhesion between corpora quadrigemina and under surface of splenium. . . . These changes had completely obliterated the vena magna

Galeni. In consequence of this obliteration there was a progressive degeneration of the plexus choroideus medianus and of the plexus choroideus lateralis up to the point where the physiologically preformed collateral path to the vena striæ terminalis admitted the formation of a collateral outlet. . . . We are not justified in assuming a stasis in the realm of the cerebro-spinal fluid, as the aqueductus Sylvii was wide, and otherwise no reason anatomically for this assumption was found."

Evidently in this case the venous compensation was either by connections with the basilar trunks resp. the suboccipital veins near their junction with the vena Galeni or by way of the infracornual veins.

5. My own case (*v. supra*, p. 42) is an excellent illustration of the effect of interference to the local venous discharge. Possibly it may be the only recorded case of obstruction limited to the straight sinus.

6. My second case (*v. supra*, p. 45) is scarcely less apposite, though the possibility of further tubercular irritation can hardly be denied.

7. J. Audry, *Revue de Médc.*, 1886, No. 11, Case I. Man of forty-five years. No tubercular or other meningeal trouble. On incising the border of the tentorium a large quantity of clear fluid escaped. In the left ventricle, attached to the choroid plexus, above the thalamus was a mobile tumor the size of a small nut. No apparent compression of thalamus or ventricular walls. He classes the fluid as an intense ventricular hydrocephalus, due to serious interference with the vascular circulation of the plexus.

8. Ransom, *Lancet*, July 1, 1893, p. 15. Man of twenty-three years. Lived for a month after onset of symptoms.

"The lateral ventricles were distended with fluid to twice their normal size. . . . The foramina of Munro were much enlarged, as was also the fourth ventricle. On the velum interpositum there was a patch of firm, fibrous thickening the size of a three-penny piece, apparently obstructing the veins of Galen."

In tumors of the cerebellum, or pressure from the posterior fossa, any attendant hydrocephalus is usually attributed to compression of this vein. In reality it may as well be due to like action on the aqueduct. Both factors doubtless combine. But that vein obstruction alone may suffice is shown by the cases given. It is, however, probable that this produces only a moderate hydrocephalus.

It is quite possible that the fluid from venous stasis here carries formed elements or precipitable fibrin that stops the ultimate absorbents. The recent observations of Wentworth (*Bost. M. and S. J.*, August 6 and 13, 1896) show that the fluid from inflammatory processes differs from the normal by its invariable cloudiness. This was due to a finely divided sediment suspended in the fluid and found to consist of mono- and polynuclear cells. After standing for a few hours it contained more or less fibrin, evidently of inflammatory origin. Quincke reports similar findings as frequent in so-called meningitis serosa.

But as already indicated, the collection of fluid from venous stasis may well be dependent on relative insufficiency of the ultimate absorbents ; and either way, the balloon-valve principle plays, secondarily at least, an important part in this form.

In cases of closure of the sinus rectus, Galen's vein or the velars, three possible outcomes are to be thought of :

1. Full physiological compensation.

2. An increase of ventricular fluid, leading to hydrocephalus.

3. Early death.

1. PERFECT COMPENSATION.

There appears to be no evidence to show that this can occur.

2. HYDROCEPHALUS.

The ample anastomoses above described, and the fact that normally this venous current has to turn several sharp angles before leaving the skull, make it, at first, unintelligible why there should ever be any trouble following the closure of the sinus rectus or its practical extension, the single trunk of Galen's vein. And, *so far as concerns either the vitality of the tissues or the function of the brain- and nerve-substance proper, there is nothing to show that compensation is less perfect than where other brain-veins are closed.*

The difference depends entirely on the presence, in the territory of this vein, of a peculiar structure, the choroidal tissue, occurring only in the brain-ventricles. This tissue normally produces ventricular fluid. Its activity is easily influenced by many conditions, and it responds quite naturally to any interference with the venous discharge by an increased production of fluid.

It is, then, not primarily any venous stasis that causes symptoms, but only the secondary hydrocephalus. And the facts show that this is always bound to occur. This causes death, if at all, only after a lengthy period and in this indirect manner.

3. EARLY DEATH.

If, however, the velars are closed (*i.e.*, the venæ intimæ be cut off from the regular outlet and from the collaterals mentioned on page 68), then, so far as present evidence goes, a speedy fatal ending is inevitable. This takes place before there is time for the development of much hydrocephalus, a small quantity of blood-tinged fluid being all that has accumulated.

Up to 1884 the writer was able to collect three such American cases ("Veins of Brain," p. 74), and those from foreign sources were merely corroborative.

It is still possible that if only the main trunk of one or both velars was obstructed, and the thrombosis did not extend into any of their branches, the fatal ending might be delayed, but hardly for long.

TREATMENT.

In view of the unsatisfactoriness of medical remedies, even though occasionally successful, it is well to inquire specially what surgical indications can be made out, and how far they can be met. In this regard there is a considerable difference, according to the form or type. In each of these it will be necessary first to formulate some plan for making a diagnosis of the form itself. This desideratum cannot be very well met as yet, but it may be in order to suggest some of the possible ways of working it out.

The fact that numerous cases have, at one time and another, been reported in which something sudden has happened, and a full cure resulted, is a further incentive on the surgical side.

Direct puncture of the brain (said by Keen to date back to the case of Dean Swift in 1744), or aspiration of the ventricles, is a very crude, inadequate, and unsatisfactory procedure. Relief is but temporary, and the danger of inducing a meningitis is increased by prolonging the drainage. This is the general verdict, and of itself the method does little towards re-establishing normal conditions.

And yet Boenninghaus (*l. c.*) has been able to collect four cases, including one of his own (three of serous and one of slightly cloudy fluid), that were cured in this way. Moreover, in infants it can be practised through an angle of the fontanelle without trephining.

Wherever a trial lumbar puncture shows pus, germs, retained blood, or any coarse products of inflammation, it is not to be expected that incisive measures will avail.

1. Where the collection is due to an impaired outflow from the fourth ventricle

What clinical evidence can we secure to show that a given case is of this type?

On spinal puncture we shall find the fluid there under only ordinary pressure (merely nominal). We shall fail to secure more than the normal surplus or residual quantity there retained (shown on page 58 to be in adults one to one and a half ounces), and, finally, what we obtain is perfectly limpid, clear cerebro-spinal fluid minus floating particles, essentially free from formed elements. A microscopical and brief chemical examination of the fluid obtained by such trial-puncture is necessary.

There may also be increased spinal reflexes, due, perhaps, to pressure of the fluid on the inhibitory tracts.

Various casual matters in individual cases may furnish additional clues.

As yet these seem to be the only determining marks that we have.

Here lumbar puncture is absolutely useless, if not decidedly injurious, except, of course, for diagnostic purposes. In these cases, be the obstruction at Magendie's foramen or at any point above, it is clear that the sacculated fluid will not be reached, but only given (by reduction of counter-resistance) a more favorable opportunity to increase locally.

The method has been found particularly dangerous in cerebellar growths, quite likely by allowing more direct mechanical action on the centres in the floor of the fourth ventricle.

But there is here a legitimate field for surgical effort. An opening should be effected in the occluding tissue,—not simply a slit made, but a good hole cut out. This need involve no hemorrhage beneath the dura. It should aim to re-establish (antochthonous) drainage. There is a question whether perfectly normal paths would be secured even in this way. Apparently, an unnatural opening would be left between subarachnoid and subdural spaces. Practically, this can be neglected.

It is certain that if there be cerebellar tumors, the same fatal termination will, without great care, follow as has occurred from spinal puncture. This and the necessity for establishing but slow and, if possible, intra-arachnoidal drainage are the most serious features of the operation.

Something of the sort has already been done in England. Alfred Parkin, of Hull (*Lancet*, 1893, ii. pp. 21 and 1244), on September 13, 1892, operated a case of tubercular meningitis by trephining the occipital bone in the median line, opening through the dura and lifting the cerebellar border so as to free the passage beneath. But, despite relief, this soon ended fatally. Later he did a successful case in a child of fourteen months. "The horse-hair drain was removed eighteen days after the operation, no fluid having come away for three days before its removal!" A diagram of the part to operate is given. He provides for gradual withdrawal of fluid by first lifting the edge of cerebellum enough to let out a little fluid only, and then draining by a few strands of silk or the like.

As he says, "Whether the openings between the fourth ventricle and the subarachnoid space are patent or not, they can easily be made so."

Lawson, *l. c.*, in his case also drained the fourth ventricle per occiput, but too freely, and death ensued in a few hours.

Ord and Waterhouse, *Lancet*, 1894, i. p. 597. "A Case, diagnosed as Tubercular Meningitis, treated by Trephining and Drainage of the Subarachnoid Space; Recovery." Girl of five years. Operated more from the side; a bent sound was then passed in on the flat, and, when opposite the occlusion, turned and used to make an opening. Drain-tube left in for eighteen days.

Glynn and Thomas, of Liverpool, *Lancet*, 1895, ii. p. 1106. "Case of Hydrocephalus; Trephining; Opening the Fourth Ventricle; Recovery." In this case, "something towards the fourth ventricle" was ruptured by finger. Man of eighteen years. Symptoms one and a half years. Drain-tube removed on the fourth day.

These English operators have made an admirable advance. But many details of the method and the extent of its applicability remain yet to be worked out.

2. Where the obstruction is in or between the ventricles.

Points for differential diagnosis of this type from the preceding are lacking. Of course, the results of a trial lumbar puncture will be the same as though the block was at Magendie's foramen. And the state of the spinal reflexes will hardly show a material difference.

Here it is hard to see what surgery can offer. In most of

the cases the retention is due to morbid growths, and the treatment becomes that of the causal trouble. In other cases there is a chance, according to Boenninghaus's statistics, of effecting a cure by direct brain puncture and withdrawal of fluid.

From his figures, it appears that about one case in six, taken as they come, has yielded a cure, but there is no evidence that the cases were of this class.

3. The irritative or inflammatory form, also that due to compression of the venous discharge from the ventricles, and apparently many congenital cases (all included under the form *e*, of p. 63).

In these the fluid-accumulation reaches, of course, down the spinal sac (subarachnoidal).   Hence a trial-puncture (lumbar) may show a higher pressure of the fluid,—and Quincke notes that this is common in meningitis serosa. We can also get more than the normal reserve quantity ; and the fluid itself, at least in the inflammatory form, will, according to Wentworth,* show even microscopically floating particles and corresponding slight turbidity.

Whether the like holds for the form due exclusively to venous stasis has not been shown, but presumably it may. The result of Quincke's injections in living animals showed, pretty conclusively, that fine suspended material is sufficient to block the ultimate absorbents.

Where trial-puncture gives fluid that is turbid or contains inflammatory products, the arachnoidal form is probable.

---

* Previously to him Huguenin had proposed similar distinguishing marks (physical and chemical), but their value has been generally disputed. Possibly a fluid, at first showing these, may gradually settle itself clear, resp. carry them along to block up the outlets, and be replaced by normal fluid.

Cultures or examinations for infective germs are proper, though rarely giving positive results in chronic cases. A chemical examination also (*v. supra*, special article by Bartley) may give further aid in diagnosis.

In this form, as the spinal centres are subjected to direct pressure by the fluid, we may expect to find the corresponding reflexes weakened, or not increased.

In congenital and early forms the presence of a spina bifida indicates arachnoidal rather than central retention.

Here the first measure to be thought of is lumbar puncture. Even in such cases, however, this is not a radical measure, and rarely gives more than symptomatic relief.

In all this class there is evidently, as indicated above, a clogging up of the arachno-absorbents. Occasionally in recent cases we might have some clearing out of these, just as we get an increased absorption after tapping a pleurisy, or by a letting up of the balloon-valve if that principle holds. But in most cases the trouble has lasted so long that the interference has become permanent.

In the acute form the causal trouble (where, as a rule, a tubercular meningitis) is the main thing, and the effusion merely a sequel of scant moment.

Simple opening of the cerebral dura has, according to Boenninghaus (*l. c.*, p. 65), been successful in four cases,— one, however, supposed to have been only a subdural cyst. Such slitting of the dura has, Boenninghaus thinks, the same action as lumbar puncture. But, as it gives such a free vent to the fluid, it represents a much more radical method. The indications therefore, however, are almost identical with those for spinal puncture considered as a remedial operation.

7

The following case illustrates well this method of procedure :

On April 28, 1897, I was asked by Dr. William Maddren to see a boy of two and a half years. The child had been brought up on the bottle, entirely so after the first six weeks of infancy. Ancestry healthy. One other child, a girl of nearly five years, is healthy,—except that she is over-stout and has a large head (fifty-three centimetres in maximum circumference).

The boy had been well and robust up to two months ago. At that time he had an attack of night-terrors, fever, and convulsions. Since then he has eaten poorly, been more restless, not slept as quietly, and in playing about the floor has shown a peculiar fear of all small objects (as feathers, fur, dust, etc.), calling them mice. Twice during this period he vomited a little mucus.

Two weeks ago he had a slight fall, striking the back and left side of the head. There was, however, no visible injury. He ran about after this, but the same day towards night his left leg gave out. This disappeared, but recurred intermittently afterwards, especially towards evening. These two weeks he has been steadily failing, has an irregular fever, once reaching 103+°, objects to being handled, and has vomited repeatedly. Some coughing. Cheyene-Stokes respiration the last two days. Involuntary urination. No ear-trouble.

The patient is a plump boy, with a good, healthy color. He lies in a stupor, continually turning his head from side to side and moaning. At every effort to move him he cries "Don't," but that is his only distinct utterance. The pulse varies, often ranging from 96 to 132, but is otherwise regular. Temperature 102.2° in rectum. No retraction of head, nor contraction of neck-muscles, except that he resists everything.

Tache cérébrale is well marked on stroking chest. Respiratory sounds normal. Splenic dulness six and a half centimetres long. Abdomen not retracted. Epigastric and abdominal reflexes present. Knee-jerks doubtful or absent. Left leg resists less than right, and only the left can be well flexed on the abdomen. Pupils wide even on illumination. Photophobia. Retinæ both show a good pink ; but the vessels are not clear, the disks are almost obscured, and the right one shows faint, pale streaking. Maximum circumference of head fifty-two and a half centimetres. No indentation or peculiarity about head, barring a slight frontal prominence of the hydrocephalic type.

Various efforts at relief had failed. Medication effected nothing and counter-irritation was unavailing. Whether the primary trouble was a tubercular meningitis could not be definitely determined. But in view of the evidence of increased intracranial pressure it was decided to try surgical measures.

Operation by Dr. Maddren, April 29. The boy was comatose at this time and fast approaching the end. The usual preparatory measures and antiseptic precautions were of course practised. A circular flap was made with base upward and apex just over the foramen magnum. In this way the field is clear to cut through to the foramen (as has been done), and yet the larger occipital arteries are avoided. There was no great amount of hemorrhage ; some spurting vessels were caught up, but no ligatures were needed.

On second removal of trephine there was a rush of clear fluid from upper part of trephine groove. A considerable quantity of fluid promptly flowed off, though only enough was caught for a bacteriological examination.* The current soon took on a pulsatory character. A somewhat freer slit was made in the dura. The button was also pried up sufficiently to run the rongeur under and chip out a small tongue of bone as a guarantee of more prolonged drainage.

A few strands of waxed silk were laid across the little bone-opening and brought out beneath the flap for a drain. Later, it was necessary to insert a tube instead, as the flap pressed down so tightly.

At the moment of first relief of tension the patient's condition became bad, but the usual restorative methods soon improved him. Only about a drachm of chloroform was used altogether. On coming out from the anæsthetic he was brighter and in better shape than at the start. By evening he revived considerably, said "mamma," asked for a "drink of water," and showed more consciousness than for forty-eight hours previously.

The temperature was not materially affected, though it dropped a degree for a day or more. By the end of the second day, however, the pulse, temperature, respiration, and general condition showed retrogression. Presently a conjugate deviation of the eyes developed, convulsions came on, and the temperature rose to 105°. He died on the fifth day after the operation.

Autopsy May 4. Skull thin. The coronal suture separated in removing the calvarium. Dura adherent. Slight scattered subdural hemorrhage over occipital region on right. Venous engorgement of posterior portion of both hemispheres. Partly organized greenish-yellow pus between the largest two vertex veins on the right, just at their entrance into the long sinus. This extended for an inch or more antero-posteriorly,—in part beyond the said veins. This was over the paracentral lobule, and had doubtless caused the weakness of the left leg.

The chiasm was embedded in similar greenish-yellow gelatiniform material, which extended posteriorly to middle of pons. Sylvians apparently free.

---

* This fluid was examined by Dr. Ezra H. Wilson, of the Hoagland Laboratory. He reports the absence of all germs, as shown both by cultures and by injections in guinea-pigs.

There was also a fine line of purulent material beneath arachnoid along the hippocampal fissure on either side.

The lateral ventricles were much enlarged, but contained only about an ounce of tinged fluid. Galen's vein was free except for post-mortem clot. Foramen of Munro open ; aqueduct of Sylvius of large size ; metapore also unobstructed.

There was an isolated tubercle * about the size of a small pea embedded in floor of fourth ventricle at about middle point on the right.

The intention in this case was to open through the foramen of Magendie— if found closed—into the fourth ventricle, and in this way drain off the internal hydrocephalus. But by finding free fluid sooner our purpose of relieving pressure was accomplished, and we therefore desisted from further interference. It was clearly, and as the autopsy proved, not a case of central but of arachnoidal retention. The basal lymph-cisterns (in particular the cisterna magna cerebello-oblongata) were directly tapped. This point is excellently situated for drainage, and with the least possible chance of infection from without.

Operative relief of this particular kind is one step in the right direction. It relieves pressure. But where the trouble is tubercular it cannot be classed as a radical measure. Even in the present case, however, it prolonged life for several days, which, in our experience, is more than can fairly be claimed for any other plan of treatment so far proposed.

Essentially similar was the procedure of D'Arçy Power (*Intnl. Clinics*, October, 1895) in two cases,—one (No. V.) of tubercular meningitis, the other (No. VI.) of non-tubercular ; both, however, ending fatally.

For a double reason the following case of Eskridge's ("Irrigation of the Posterior Cerebral Fossa for the Relief of Basilar Meningitis," *Jrnl. N. and M. Dis.*, November, 1895) is worth giving more fully. It was that of a man of thirty, "with the appearance of one dying from intracranial pressure." The trephine "opening was about on the level of the posterior margin of the foramen magnum, and about three-fourths of an inch to the left of the median line of

---

* In this Dr. Wilson found plenty of giant-cells and tubercle bacilli.

the occipital bone." "A large amount of cerebro-spinal fluid escaped." "A soft catheter was passed in through the opening in the dura, and the subdural spaces freely irrigated in all directions with normal salt solution. To the right of the median line the catheter easily passed, without obstruction, a distance of over two inches." Considerable improvement. Death on third day. Autopsy, "In the centrum ovale of the left frontal lobe a considerable quantity of semi-fluid blood was found, which, after ploughing up and destroying a considerable portion of this part of the brain, ruptured into the lateral ventricle and filled the lateral third and fourth ventricles. The corpora striata were softened. A slight hemorrhagic extravasation was found in the right frontal lobe. The remainder of the brain presented a normal appearance."

In looking about for other possible measures of relief, two suggest themselves. One is by making openings or communication between the subarachnoid space and the general extra-spinal resp. extra-cranial cellular tissue. But various attempts of the kind have been tried, and so far with little encouragement. It remains, however, the real desideratum. The other is by any measure that shall renew or increase the natural absorbents from the subarachnoid space. Some good will follow spinal gymnastics. By this is meant a utilization of the normal mobility of the spine, and consequent up-and-down motion of the cord therein, as well as by the attendant increase and decrease of cerebrospinal pressure. By curving the spine anteriorly all its tissues are put on the stretch and the capacity of the vertebral canal presumably is increased. By arching backward (opisthotonos) the same tissues are certainly relaxed, and the space of the vertebral canal materially diminished.

Thus a considerable pressure can be exerted towards forcing open any outlets.

In patients old enough to have sense, this exercise can be practised voluntarily. In younger ones it can be carried out passively.

Any such plan applies, of course, only to cases with free communication between the brain-accumulation and the spinal space. The good accomplished, however, will be not merely symptomatic, but tend towards radical relief. If we can diagnosticate this form, then a systematic course of the above kind, well persisted in, gives some promise of good, and is rational.

Perhaps comparable to the gymnastic forcing of exits is the plan of Locatelli, of Milan (*v. Arch. f. Pediatrics*, 1886, p. 488). He exposes the child's bare occiput to solar rays for half an hour or so daily. Later, this method was advocated by Sourma, *Deut. Medizinal Zeitung*, June 20, 1888 (*v.* Sajous's "Annual," 1889, vol. ii.), who began with only fifteen minutes' exposure.

Evidently this acts by a slow but powerful expansion of the liquid. His procedure might possibly avail in hydrocephalus cut off from the general subarachnoid, while the gymnastic plan is limited in value to such cases as are not so cut off.

XII.

PSEUDO-BULBAR PARALYSIS.

BILATERAL APOPLEXY OF THE LENTICULAR NUCLEI, SIMULATING LESION IN THE FLOOR OF THE FOURTH VENTRICLE.*

It has not been thought possible as yet to include injury of the lenticular nuclei among the forms of brain disease which admit of approximate localization. A limited number of cases have, however, accumulated which seem to indicate that an insult to both these nuclei, and perhaps to only one, may produce a picture of its own.

Since, however, these bodies are, from statistics, a very frequent seat of apoplexy, and, besides, entirely latent foci have been found in them at the autopsy, it is probable that the special symptomatology observed in the other cases was caused not by the lenticular injury itself but by an extension of it or its effects to adjacent parts. Be that as it may, that injury of these bodies may produce a very well-marked and peculiar group of symptoms is shown by the following case. It occurred in the practice of Dr. Fuller, and was seen in consultation by Dr. McNaughton. The

---

* Reprinted, with some emendations, from a paper read before the New York Neurological Society, October 7, 1884, and, conjointly with the late Dr. S. E. Fuller, published in the *New York Medical Record* of November 1, 1884.

interest of the case was fully recognized, and pains were taken to observe all symptoms. The clinical history is furnished by Dr. Fuller; the results of the autopsy and the appended remarks are by Dr. Browning.

A lady, M. J., aged sixty years, complained one day, while sewing, of sudden numbness and tingling in the left foot and ankle. Rubbing gave relief, and it passed off without any physician being called. In fact, this was very likely a local matter. Eleven months after, she was one evening attacked with a feeling of numbness in the tongue and peculiar sensations in the left side of the body. There was no aphasia nor loss of consciousness, and she was perfectly able to describe her own feelings. The most important objective symptom was a left hemiparesis. The motor weakness disappeared entirely in about two weeks. The present attack occurred without premonitions five months and a half later. It came on about four P.M., July 16, 1884, while in the bath-room. She is said to have called out to a lady in the next room, saying she was very dizzy and had pain in her head; the lady helped her to bed. There seemed to have been no loss of consciousness on the patient's part.

Upon my arrival she was speechless, and remained so. It was only possible for her to make an expiratory guttural sound. Having been paralyzed before, she immediately proceeded to show me that it was not the same by raising first the right arm and leg and then the left. The lips, tongue, and muscles of deglutition were paralyzed; the saliva flowed from whichever angle of the mouth was lowermost; the upper portion of the facial nerve was functionally intact, and the pupils reacted normally. She could not open her jaws, or only to the slightest extent. The lower jaw could be readily depressed with the finger, but on attempting to swab out collecting mucus from the oral cavity and throat—as was often necessary—the jaws would close and press on whatever had been introduced into the mouth, despite the strongest desire of the patient to keep them open. The nurse had to be instructed, before cleansing the mouth, to wrap a blade in soft material and place it edgeways, so as to keep the jaws apart until the little procedure was finished. This symptom persisted during the conscious life of the patient. The tongue was quite motionless.

The urine had been examined some time previously and found free from albumin. Immediately subsequent to this attack there was an enormously increased flow of urine. In the first three hours she passed water three times. Though not measured, it was estimated by the attendants to have been a quart each time. In this urine there was about twenty vol. per cent. of albumin and once a trace of sugar with Fehling's test. Within twenty-four hours the quantity of urine returned to normal. Albumin persisted in it, for a time at least. She snored very loudly after the attack, though not doing so previously. There was no trouble from the soft palate when awake, although it hung in a paralyzed condition.

So long as she remained conscious—*i.e.*, for the first five days—she always gave notice of a desire to defecate or urinate ; no incontinence whatever. During the same period she would often motion for spectacles, paper, and pencil, indicating that the latter be first moistened in the mouth. She would then communicate by writing her questions, and showed the full possession of her mental faculties. This was further shown by her remembering when medicine was due (given per rectum and hypodermically), by directing attention when a sample of urine had been forgotten, and in a variety of other ways,—*e.g.*, curiosity as to the nature and cause of her own condition. She would, however, cry rather easily, the tears then running silently down over the cheeks. This could hardly be wondered at or considered as loss of control over the feelings.

It is very doubtful if she succeeded in swallowing anything, though she tried hard to do so. She was successfully nourished with peptonized milk, etc., per rectum.

The sterno-cleido and other large neck muscles did not appear to be affected. The sense of hearing remained good, and, in fact, no anæsthesia of any part of the body was discovered.

The pulse, respiration, and temperature showed no disturbance to within forty-eight hours of death. At this time, after some extra exertion on her part, she gradually sank into a stupor. Some twelve hours before the end she became very much flushed and hot to the touch over the whole body. This afterwards gave place to a kind of collapse. Death on the morning of July 23.

Post-mortem in the afternoon, with the assistance of Drs. Fuller and McNaughton. The autopsy being permitted only on condition that nothing whatever be carried away, it was impossible to make a minute examination of any of the parts, yet this could not have added very materially to the exactness of the present case. Only the brain was removed, including the cord to opposite the second cervical vertebra.

The cerebro-spinal fluid was slightly increased. The vertebral and carotid arteries with their branches on the base of the brain presented numerous patches of atheroma, but were, at least in all their larger divisions, still permeable. No further abnormal appearances on any portion of the surface of the brain.

The lateral ventricles presented nothing unusual, unless some slight adhesions between the ependyma of the ventricular roof and floor. Laterally in the brain-substance, on the two sides very nearly symmetrical, were two recent clots. These were in the lenticular nuclei, extending into all three divisions and tapering off posteriorly.

On the right side, in front of and external to the recent effusion, were the remains of what must have been a considerable hemorrhage. This had extended antero-posteriorly along the external capsule, from nearly opposite the front end of the ventricle to about opposite the front end of the recent hemorrhage, and was consequently just beneath the island of Reil. The claustrum had not been broken through externally, nor the lenticular nucleus attacked internally. There was simply an oblong space remaining, with slightly separated walls enclosing a little brownish, thick fluid matter. The said walls consisted of somewhat thickened and discolored tissue without any smooth interior surface. Such is, according to Charcot, the usual form and appearance of old extravasations at this point. This had clearly caused the former left hemiplegia. Motor fibres are not known to traverse this tract. The paralysis must, therefore, have been caused by pressure transmitted from the clot, a view which is corroborated by her recovery.

As to the recent extravasations, the same general description will apply to both. Each was in amount equal, perhaps, to a pigeon's egg. The nerve-tissue was not only much torn but, from the size of the clot and its longitudinal form, also forced apart. The two were, from their appearance, of about the same date. It was not possible in either of them to distinguish any older or newer portion. They were very dark, in part semi-fluid, and, so far as color and character of the clot went, at least one or two days old, perhaps several.

The head of each clot was about opposite the front end of the thalamus, and diminished backward to nearly opposite the posterior end of the same. The main portion appeared to be wholly in the lenticular nucleus, while its posterior prolongation or branches may have encroached to a limited extent on other structures.

No further foci were found in any part of the brain. The medulla oblongata, pons, etc., presented no morbid appearance. Sections through these parts were made very close together, so that even a pin-head clot could not have escaped notice. Embolism or thrombosis of a week's standing must have produced visible softening, so that they also can be excluded. Possibly one or both the apoplectic centres were at first much smaller, and an added effusion of blood brought on the stupor of the last few days, with the fatal termination. But there was nothing in the foci to indicate this, and the time at which the final condition developed corresponds to that at which surrounding reaction and the symptoms dependent thereon so often occur. Hence the simpler explanation, that there was but one attack without further hemorrhage on either side, is at the same time the more tenable.

The recent effusions were so considerable and the tissues about them were so torn as to render them valueless for the localization of any isolated symptom. The interest of the case, however, lies in the peculiar combination of symptoms. These presented a complex believed to indicate lesion in a part that at the autopsy was found intact. To recall some of them : the paralysis was bilateral, quite symmetrical as regards both extent and severity, and occurred on the two sides simultaneously. There was no loss of consciousness. Immediately there was a greatly increased flow of urine, containing both albumin and sugar. There was also well-marked labio-glosso-pharyngeal paralysis. This forms a group of symptoms the cause of which is generally assigned to trouble in the floor of the fourth ventricle. Thrombosis or embolism of a terminal bulbar artery is credited with almost identical consequences, and apoplexy from one of the same vessels may not appear very different.

To Joffroy (1872) is given the credit of first suggesting the possible occurrence of this cerebral form. Then in 1877 Lepine followed with three actual cases that he had collected. A limited number of observations presenting various degrees of similarity to the present one are considered by Ross in his work on "Diseases of the Nervous System" (vol. ii. pp. 626–628 of first edition, continued in the second. Also two cases of depots in the lenticular nuclei— one unilateral—are given by him in *Brain* for July, 1882). From these he concludes that destruction of the lenticular nuclei in the whole or in part *may* produce nearly if not quite all the symptoms of lesion in the oblongata. His cases, however, ran a slower course, and were less typical of acute bulbar trouble. He notes that consciousness may not be lost at the occurrence of this accident, but does not in any of his cases mention disturbance in the urinary secretion.

Wernike mentions the occurrence of bulbar symptoms

in cerebral disease. He even cites a case of pseudo-bulbar paralysis where, however, the pathological conditions varied materially from that under consideration. To produce this grouping of symptoms the lenticular trouble must affect fibres in their course through the internal capsule from the cortical to the bulbar centres, or else compress cortical centres directly opposite. It is now generally accepted that the speech tract, inclusive of mouth-facial and hypoglossus, takes a somewhat distinct path through the knee of the internal capsule. In the present case the two hemorrhages must have occurred at the same time. Although not into a part vitally so important as the medulla, yet from their size and after-effects they proved fatal.

Experimental destruction of one or both of these nuclei has not established any facts available in localization. Ferrier, together with many neurologists, simply believes that hemiplegia may result from such injury when unilateral. But these cases, while not disproving, certainly do not confirm this. As to the possibility of distinguishing between these two (the cerebral and the bulbar) forms, when acute, some points may be noticed. In the present case there were no convulsions ; no paralysis below the throat ; nothing unusual in pulse or respiration ; evidently no trouble with the sense of hearing, but increased reflex excitability of the muscles of the jaw (M. J. Lewis's chin-reflex). In bulbar lesions the corresponding reflexes are, on the contrary, lowered, while the other symptoms, here absent, occur with more or less frequency. Abnormal activity of the emotional expressions of the face has been repeatedly noted in the cerebral cases.

Such and similar points of discrimination would, however, in view of the very limited number of known cases from which to draw conclusions, hardly warrant confidence in an attempt at differential diagnosis.

The occurrence of trismus as a symptom in brain-lesions is treated by W. von Hanger in the *Wien. Med. Wchr.*, 1886, No. 5. Although in bulbar lesions the corresponding reflexes are often impaired, this does not always hold, for Miles (*Arch. of Medc.*, August, 1882) has published a case of hemorrhage in the floor of the fourth ventricle, where for months there was a tonic contraction of the muscles of mastication, and hence with increased reflex-excitability of the same.

Many writers acknowledge the lack of distinguishing critera between the false and the true form of bulbar paralysis. Further, it has become evident that, exclusive of the asthenic form, in which no changes are found, these cases of the pseudo-type are very varied in their pathology ; few are as simple and symmetrical as the above.

XIII.

A CASE OF SYMMETRICALLY SITUATED DOUBLE HEMOR-RHAGE OF THE BRAIN.[*]

CASE of Mrs. ——, aged thirty-nine years. No previous history, except the existence of an ulcer of the left leg, for about ten years off and on, which at the time of her admission into the hospital was the size of a man's palm, deep, and offensive in odor. The left leg was swollen below the knee, œdematous and discolored ; foot also œdematous. Five weeks before admission into the hospital the patient complained to her niece of "general debility" and a "weakness" especially of left side of body, and also of a severe headache in the right parietal region, which was pretty constant, and was described as if her head "was a hollow iron pot with some one hammering inside."

Upon the morning of her admission into the hospital she got up feeling pretty well, but soon began to drop things from her left hand. Then her leg began to get weak. But she went herself and made application for entrance into the hospital. While being conveyed from the central office (about two P.M.) by wagon, in getting in or out, she fell once, and had to be helped to her feet, but walked fairly well after that.

When seen by the hospital physician, about three o'clock

---

[*] Reported by Mark Manley, A.B., M.D., late of the house-staff of the King's County Hospital.

P.M., June 12, 1896, she sat up all right, but could not walk
without assistance.   There were muscular twitchings of the
left arm and leg, with a sensation as of "pins and needles"
in the left side of body, principally in the arm and leg, and
especially in the sole of the left foot.   The arm could then
be used somewhat, but the leg not as well.   The left lower
facial was paretic,—as shown by the mouth being drawn to
the right in smiling.   No pupillary changes nor disturbance
of the motor oculi.

Next seen about five-thirty o'clock P.M.   Patient was
then practically comatose.   The left arm and leg were in
continual tetanic contraction.   There were some spasmodic
(apparently) movements of the left hand.   The head and
eyes rotated to the right.   There was partial ptosis of right
eye, and possibly slight ptosis of left also.   Vomiting was
continuous and projectile in character.   Right pupil was
dilated and external strabismus marked ; pulse very weak.

The patient continued in this condition for three days
until she died.   The vomiting stopped after the first few
hours.

The autopsy on brain, about three days after death,
was by Dr. Browning, in whose service the case occurred.   The brain had been removed shortly after death,
and thus some of its relations had been rendered uncertain.   On the base no morbid alterations were apparent,
and no atheromatous patches were to be seen in the vessels.
On the right hemisphere there was an extensive discolora-
tion and bulging in the mid- and supra-parietal region.
There was a couple of spots here where the hemorrhage
had ground through the cortex and just appeared subpial,
but not to the extent of more than a considerable external
suffusion.   The discolored region was two inches or more

8

across, though irregular. It lacked a scant inch of reaching to the superior border. Below it extended to about
the level of the juncture of the inferior and middle thirds
of the central region. There was no effusion into the
ventricles. There was a vast lesion on the right. Under
the motor region was an extensive hemorrhage, and
chowdering of brain-substance. The bulk of the hemorrhage was under the junction of the middle and upper
thirds of the central region. The condition of the broken-
up tissue suggested previous changes in it, but not with
certainty. The outer portion of the thalamus was involved
in the comminution. Anterior to but continuous with this
was another collection of blood and broken-up tissue. The
lenticular nucleus and structures between this and the surface of insula were pretty well disintegrated and mixed with
blood.

A large part of the caudate nucleus showed grayish-
yellow softening, almost like pus, evidently antedating the
hemorrhage. From about the anterior extremity of the
lenticular nucleus, and extending into the white substance
of the anterior lobe, was a collection of pale yellowish
fluid (indefinite cyst, resp. remains of some former trouble).
This was immediately adjacent to and forward of the anterior extremity of the hemorrhage.

On the opposite or left side of the brain there was no
visible change externally. But on making sections, many
punctiform hemorrhages (the little coagula could be readily
separated with the knife) were found through the substance
of the upper extremity of the central convolutions, and
even a little posteriorly to same. From this point these
hemorrhages occurred in a downward and forward direction, rather crossing to the front of the central convolu-

tions, and finally ceasing about opposite their middle point. Midway in this tract of hemorrhages was one larger and longer up and down, amounting in its whole volume to the size of a large pea. This belt of fine hemorrhages on the left was directly opposite to—*i.e.*, corresponded in position with—the main volume of hemorrhage on the right. No trace of hemorrhage elsewhere on left side.

In the cerebral crura, pons, oblongata, cerebellum, neighboring vessels, etc., no macroscopic change was found, even on section. The basilar vessels, however, were not in shape to admit of much examination.

In this case the initial symptoms show that the hemorrhage started in the region where the greatest effusion was found. That in such a case, with a person only thirty-nine years of age and still free from marked atheroma, we should find a great number of minute hemorrhages, and at least one somewhat larger, and all these limited to a narrow belt quite symmetrical with the primary and main effusion, is striking in the extreme. This, doubtless, might have been overlooked had we not been on the watch for it. The fact that they were so numerous showed some peculiar influence acting on that region,—an influence that affected many or all the small vessels.

XIV.

ON DOUBLE (SYNCHRONOUS AND SYMMETRICAL) HEMOR-
RHAGES OF THE BRAIN.

It has long been evident that there were some points in the pathology of cerebral hemorrhage not yet worked out, —that the whole matter was not summed up in the existence of aneurisms, miliary or otherwise. For a small proportion of cases it is shown, in another chapter, that areas of softening are responsible. Some further grounds indicating the incompleteness of this old explanation of Charcot and Bouchard are as follows :

A. The not rare onset during sleep, a time when certainly we should expect least strain on vessel-walls. It is to be remembered that often a subconjunctival and even a nasal hemorrhage likewise occurs during sleep, and, moreover, without the intervention of any known aneurism.

B. Constipation and intestinal disorders in some way favor its occurrence. This is in certain cases noticeable independent of any straining at stool. In the older literature, here and there, is a case where apoplexy was brought into relation with biliary or renal calculi, or some special abdominal disturbance, the pain element, apparently, not being the factor.

C. It is surprising that epileptic convulsions so rarely cause vascular rupture. Though many such cases have been reported, yet it still remains a very unusual occurrence, and is so regarded by the authorities (R. Reynolds, Harbinson, Niemeyer, etc.).

D. The frequent occurrence of prodromata. These are largely ignored in discussions, and are certainly often absent or unrecognized. They have been explained on the basis of a supposed inaugural oozing before full rupture, but such a view it is difficult to appreciate. As they precede the seizure by so short a period, they cannot well be attributed to any irritative effect of the aneurisms. Perhaps as yet they have not been brought into sufficiently close relation to hemorrhagic apoplexy by post-mortem proof. In the absence of this last, it is still possible that these were really cases of thrombosis.

E. The careful work of numerous observers has shown that in many of these cases no aneurisms can be found, and, even if present, are not necessarily the source of the effusion.

F. Moreover, scattered through the literature of the subject are various cases of bilateral and fairly symmetrical hemorrhages developing at nearly or quite the same time. The reason why more are not on record is, evidently, the simple one that nobody has thought to look specially for them, the effusion on one side being usually of such a minor character as to escape notice. Besides, of late years single lesions chiefly have been published, as they better serve for purposes of localization.

This last point (*F*) carries with it a possible solution of the whole query.

The term "symmetrical" is here used to indicate the point of departure of the bleeding, and not necessarily its size or shape. Inasmuch as the two hemispheres of any brain are not perfectly symmetrical, and still less the vessels

of the two sides, it follows that physiologically corresponding points may not have quite the same site. This merely
allows a little more latitude in the interpretation of cases.

So far as present argument goes, these foci may be either
strictly "synchronous" or immediately consecutive the one
to the other.

While it is not unusual to find remains of multiple old
hemorrhages at autopsy, such cases can hardly be utilized
here. Even in the rather frequent cases where they are
found symmetrical, the history of their development is so
far lacking that it is impossible to say whether they were
synchronous in origin or not.

1. Case of double lenticular hemorrhage, *v. supra*, p. 103.

2. Woman of twenty-one years, admitted to Kings County
Hospital September 20, 1895. Three months pregnant.
Dysentery. Very delirious. Later, quiet but entirely irra-
tional. Death in a day or two. The autopsy (by Dr. Van
Cott, who kindly called my attention to the matter) showed
"hemorrhage in anterior part of both corpora striata and
posterior portion of right thalamus."

3. Case reported above, p. 112.

4. Andral, Obs. 15. Man of seventy-two years. For some
time said to have frequently swooned. The day before,
the faint had been more prolonged. Admitted in profound coma. Death, without change, in about a week.

At junction of posterior and middle thirds of right hemisphere, an inch below the superior surface, was a clot the
size of a hazel-nut. An equal-sized clot similarly situated
in left hemisphere. (More fully given in Wernicke, Bd. ii.
p. 88.)

5. Charcot and Bouchard, *Arch. de Physiol. Norm. et
Pathol.*, 1868, p. 644, Case III. of recent hemorrhages.

Woman of seventy-four years. Apoplexy. Coma. Resolution of extremities perhaps greater on right side than on the left, but without manifest predominance of the paralysis on either side. Death same day. In the left hemisphere a large effusion had ploughed up the substance of the centrum ovale and torn the striated body. Another effusion a little less voluminous existed in the symmetrical points of the right hemisphere.

There was also a small focus in the pons and a further one in the left cerebral crus. Miliary aneurisms in the convolutions. Kidneys large but unaltered in structure.

6. Ollivier, *Gaz. hebd.*, 1875 (*v.* Wernicke, vol. ii. p. 45). Man of seventy-five years. Sudden attack. Coma. Death in thirty-two hours. A fresh hemorrhage in the centre of each thalamus : on the left, the size of a hazel-nut; on the right, of a small pea. A smaller hemorrhage in the pons.

7. A. Harbinson, *Jrnl. Mental Sci.*, October, 1877, p. 356. Epileptic, insane female of thirty-six years. A condition of mental torpor followed some severe seizures. Death a day later. "Symmetrically situated in each postero-parietal lobule was an apoplexy the size of a walnut, containing in its centre several separate and distinct soft, recent clots (three on the left and five or six on the right), from the size of a pea to that of a cherry. In the third left occipital convolution was another clot, the size and shape of an almond, splitting up the white fibres ; and in the second left temporo-sphenoidal was a rather smaller one." Other changes.

8. P. Richer, *Bull. Soc. Anat. de Paris*, Février, 1878, p. 94. Attack of apoplexy with loss of consciousness. Right hemiplegia with contractures. Death from pneumonia four

years later.   Old double hemorrhage in central part of each hemisphere.   Pediculo-frontal section on left showed the striate body, including lenticular and caudate nuclei and intervening internal capsule destroyed.   On the other side was a linear hemorrhagic focus between the external capsule (which was intact) and the lenticular nucleus.

9. Charcot et Pitres, *Arch. de Med.*, May, 1883, Case XL. (from M. H. Blaise, 1882).   Man of seventy-four years. Attack with loss of consciousness for half an hour.   After the apoplectic state had passed no motor or sensory trouble could be made out.   At evening the next day he was carried off by a pulmonary congestion without having presented any paralytic phenomena.

In the right hemisphere was a capillary hemorrhage size of a five-franc piece, occupying the upper part of the parieto-occipital fissure, extending out a little on its superior portion.   In the left hemisphere an anologous focus above the interparietal fissure and in the posterior middle of the superior parietal lobule.

10. L. Löwenfeld, "Ätiologie und Pathogenese der spontanen Hirnblutungen," Wiesbaden, 1886, Case XIV.   Man of fifty-eight years.   "Multiple old cysts, probably in part of hemorrhagic origin (with yellowish-red pigmented walls), and fresh foci of softening in the insular region on both sides and in the left parietal lobe."   He gives this under "Sitz des Blutherdes," on p. 35.   Then, on p. 84, referring to the same case, he says that in the wall of the focus several ruptured vessels (without aneurisms) were found that were connected with blood-coagula.

While this description is not complete, it seems to indicate fresh hemorrhages of the insulæ, and hence symmetrical.

11. Allen Sym, *Edinburgh Med. Jrnl.*, November, 1890, pp. 468, 469. Young woman, aged twenty-two years. Ill about ten days ; bilious vomiting, with unconscious jerking of limbs, etc., later. The brain showed multiple hemorrhages in the optic thalami, besides an excess of fluid in the lateral ventricles.

12. Hebold, *Arch. f. Psychiatrie*, 1892, Bd. xxiii., "Herderkrankungen im Putamen des Linsenkernes," p. 451. His second case. Widow of eighty-two years. In the left lenticular nucleus against the claustrum was a hemorrhagic softening, and the same in less extent on the other side.

13. Eskridge's case, *v. supra*, p. 101.

Perhaps a peculiar observation of C. K. Mills (*Phila. Med. Times*, 1879, vol. ix. p. 269) belongs here : "In regard to the occurrence of lesions in both corpora striata, I might say that I have several times seen cysts or softening in one of the basal ganglia, apparently formed subsequently to a lesion of the corresponding body on the other side of the brain."

And very striking are the rare cases of symmetrical porencephalic defect. Audry (*Rev. de Médc.*, 1888, pp. 462 and 553) notes that of ninety-six well-described cases of porencephalia, thirty-two presented lesions in both hemispheres and were then always symmetrical. And he does not seem to include the like case of Bianchi (*v. Am. Jrnl. Nrlg. and Pschty.*, 1884, p. 622). Some of these were due to other causes, as specific arteritis, emboli, etc.

The number of cases here presented may be small, yet is sufficient to bring up certain queries and considerations.

1. Are these really symmetrical ?

For most of the cases this is so nearly if not absolutely

true that their symmetrical character cannot well be questioned.

2. Are these mere coincidences?

So far as those collected from other sources go this might possibly be claimed, although any careful search of the literature would give further support to the existence of such a class. But my own cases have been sufficiently convincing to negative any such supposition.

Where in any given case one point gives way there may well be numerous other spots in the same brain almost equally weak. Hence it might not be so surprising to occasionally meet with a double rupture. But it is remarkable that, of the comparatively few cases in which a double effusion develops at the same time, such a considerable number should be symmetrical. In view of the large extent of the brain, this is too much to be explained by any theory of chances.

3. Can the two be due to any general or systemic state?

Hardly, for neither, then, would their location be opposite and symmetrical.

Symmetrical embolisms, aneurisms, and even tumors of the brain have in rare instances been observed. But such occurrences have no apparent bearing on the present question. More common are correspondingly situated bilateral foci of softening. And as these, especially involving the central ganglia, are occasionally due to toxic influences, it is just possible that some similar cause might produce symmetrical hemorrhages. There is, however, no further evidence in support of such a supposition. And cases of hemorrhage following infectious diseases, so far as recorded, fail to show any such bilateralism.

4. Are there any local changes or dynamic conditions that might suffice for an explanation?

The supposition of a direct mechanical cause like contrecoup, or of double focussing like the acoustics of an echochamber, loses force when we recall that these hemorrhages are not diagonally but directly opposite.

According to Todd (*Lond. Med. Gaz.*, 1850, p. 780), it was first pointed out by Bizot that it was quite common for the arteries of the brain to be diseased in a symmetrical manner. But if there is anything in this, it, doubtless, refers to the main arterial trunks,* and these are rarely the seat of rupture. Even if disease of these smaller vessels were bilateral, that does not explain why both should give way together.

Possibly the reason why these double hemorrhages are not more common or striking is that, to produce large effusions, some change in both the symmetrical vessels, favoring rupture, must be present.

5. Such peculiar relation of the hemorrhages may, evidently, occur in any part of the cerebrum. At least, these cases show no special preference for any region,—except for those parts more frequently the site of hemorrhage, five out of thirteen involving the central ganglia,—though none were in the cerebellum or pons oblongata. In the pons it is not so unusual to find a hemorrhage reaching across to both sides, but presumably it has originated from a single point.

---

* Hadden (*Trans. Pathol. Soc.*, London, 1884, vol. xxxv. p. 73) gives a case of "Symmetrical Aneurisms of the Middle Cerebral Arteries," occurring where the perforantes are given off. One of these had so ruptured as to cause an effusion into the substance of the brain. S. West, *ibid.*, 1889–90, vol. xli. p. 59, gives another case : vessels thin ; no cause for the aneurisms found. And W. H. White, *ibid.*, pp. 60–62, gives such a case, with symptoms resembling cerebro-spinal meningitis.

6. There must be some common, mutual, or interdependent influence that effects this symmetry. The only explanation left is that this depends on nerve action, most probably vaso-motor.

That there may be a bilateral coördination in the innervation of the brain-arteries is in no sense strange, though it has hardly been recognized heretofore. But that a purely nervous influence plays a direct part in the development of hemorrhagic apoplexy presents a new principle in cerebral pathology.*

Even though one focus is primary and the other secondary thereto, it still shows that brain-hemorrhage may be produced by nervous influence, and thus quite as perfectly puts this factor on an established basis.

The full significance of the principle can be worked out but slowly ; and many more or less speculative queries immediately arise.

That it indicates the cause of the premonitory focal symptoms observed in some cases of hemorrhage—viz., a preliminary vascular paralysis—is pointed out in another chapter.

Where one of the effusions remains small, it may occasionally, at the autopsy, serve to localize more definitely the starting-point of the major bleeding.

An important question here is whether any other form of nerve-influence than vaso-motor could accomplish or explain this occurrence ? This seems improbable, though it cannot quite be denied.

---

* Löwenfeld, *l. c.*, p. 145, says, " Positive evidence of the participation of a nervous factor [in the causation of brain-hemorrhage] is not as yet at hand ; we are only in position to cite a series of circumstances that speak for such an influence."

In his recent work on the "Cerebral Circulation" (London, 1896), L. Hill, after detailing numerous experiments that he has tried, says he has "been entirely unable to find any evidence of a vaso-motor supply to the brain," p. 45. After considering his own results and the work of others, he concludes, p. 75 : "The brain has no direct vaso-motor mechanism, but its blood-supply can be controlled indirectly by the vaso-motor centre acting on the splanchnic area. . . . There is, undoubtedly, muscular tissue in the vessels of the pia mater, and it may well be asked, Why is this muscle present if it does not constrict? Gulland [in a recent and exhaustive research] has entirely failed to demonstrate vaso-motor nerves in the vessels of the pia. The muscle is an elastic, supporting structure capable of withstanding internal tension, but as far as the principles of the cerebral circulation are in question it may otherwise be neglected. If there is constriction or dilatation of the cerebral vessels, it is so small that it is overcome passively by any rise in the general pressure."

Such wholesale ignoring of the muscular structure in the brain-arteries cannot be allowed any weight, and can, certainly, convince no one who has ever examined these vessel-walls microscopically. Even on theoretical grounds it cannot stand. The brain-veins have lost their muscular element, owing (as was pointed out by the writer in 1884, and is amply verified by the work of Hill himself) to the fact that they are merely passive elastic tubes. It was impossible for the relatively weak veins to exert any independent action where all the conditions of pressure were dictated by the stronger arteries. Hence the muscular layer in these veins has completely dropped out. If now the arteries were in their turn completely secondary to some controlling force outside the cranium (as Hill contends), then they also must long ere this have discarded their muscular layer likewise. But the fact that the layer is still present proves the contrary. And if so, it must be under some control. Because experiments do or do not find proof of a vaso-motor supply to the brain cannot, for an instant, impugn the necessary fact that some control does exist.

Hill's conclusion has already been attacked by Obersteiner (Wien, 1897, *v. Neurlgc. Centbl.*, 1897, p. 356), who succeeded in demonstrating nerves in the smaller arteries of the pia.

7. How is this influence exercised? Do both effusions start together (one common preceding influence), or does one soon induce the other?

Though the evidence on this point is far from decisive, it rather indicates that the former supposition is the correct one.

a. It is not necessary that either be very large.

b. Yet it seems to be only about the starting-point that the two correspond. In Case III. the secondary focus remained limited and did not spread commensurably with the first. Certainly any correlation of the sides soon ceases.

c. The result of the experiments (*v.* pp. 39–41) points negatively in the same direction.

d. This view suffices better to clear up the points raised at the outset of this paper.

8. Is this influence (vaso-motor) sufficient of itself to produce leakage or rupture of brain-vessels? Apparently it is, although to produce any large effusion there very likely must be some previous alteration in the vessel-walls favoring rupture.

9. The multiple character of one or both foci in Cases III., VII., and XI., and perhaps IX. and X., suggests a special form distinct from the general run of apoplexies. It, however, proves that, occasionally at least, not some single point but a considerable stretch of vessel is at fault. This serves to more fully corroborate the fact that morbid vaso-motor action is at the bottom of the trouble. The possibility of an encephalitis hemorrhagica is negatived by the facts.

The punctate hemorrhages frequently observed after brain-shock may on this basis be a secondary neuro-effect (as the anæmia has been shown to be), and not a direct result of the violence.

The main principle involved in the explanation is just as fully demonstrated, even though these cases prove to be but a special class.

10. Cases in which this form does not occur.

As a rule, it does not in those due to rupture of meningeal vessels, or to traumatism, whether in the meninges or in the substance of the brain, or to syphilitic disease of the arteries, or to softening (absent in one such case specially examined therefor, *v*. p. 129, Case II., though another case, *v*. p. 114, makes this questionable).

It remains to be determined how frequently, in the remaining ordinary spontaneous cases, some trace of this, ranging from simply dilated arteries to punctate and larger hemorrhages, does occur.

XV.

NOTE ON THE OCCURRENCE OF BRAIN-HEMORRHAGE STARTING IN A FOCUS OF SOFTENING.

To the causes of cerebral hemorrhage should be added —more definitely, at least, than has yet been done—the pre-existence of spots of softening. Presumably these arrode, or at least implicate and weaken, the wall of some vessel in the involved area ; then follows the rupture. It is not material to the pathology of such a case whether some aneurismal dilatation has developed as an intermediary or not.

A brief outline of two cases of this kind may suffice to call attention to the matter.

1. The subject was a man thirty-seven years of age, just recovering from some ill-defined trouble. Severe apoplectic seizure. Death within twenty-four hours. Autopsy in December, 1888, with Dr. McNaughton and the late Dr. Fuller.

There was a large hemorrhage starting from a small area of softening to the outer side of the left post-cornu. This had not chowdered the brain-substance, but promptly broken into the horn. Owing to this ready outlet into the ventricle the antecedent softening was, in this case, practically undisturbed, and hence unmistakable. It was made up of a diffluent, brownish material, but slightly mixed with blood. Had this been deeper in the hemisphere, the

128

bleeding must have burrowed and ground up surrounding brain-substance sufficient to have obscured the primary focus.

The blood had filled the left lateral, passed through the foramen of Munro to some extent into the right lateral, but principally by way of the third ventricle and the iter into the fourth. From this it had oozed out on either side subarachnoidal. A little had also passed out per metapore.

2. The second case was in a brain that I examined through the courtesy of Dr. Van Cott, in October, 1896. It was from a woman who had died two hours after admission to the Long Island College Hospital.

There had been a most extensive effusion of blood. It had scattered out generally under the arachnoid of both hemispheres, but collected in largest amount in the cisternæ about the base. A careful hunt for the source showed that it came from a subpial focus of softening, about two centimetres in diameter, on the median surface of the tip of the left frontal lobe. The pre-existing detritus was unmistakable, and the open vessel beside it. There were no hemorrhagic specks nor especially dilated vessels in the corresponding part of the right frontal lobe, though there was a smaller spot of broken-down tissue in the anterior part of the right insula.

If in this case the spot of softening had been deeper in the hemisphere, then the amount of brain-tissue torn up in such position by the hemorrhage itself must easily have masked previous disintegration. But the immediate outlet, after rupture of the artery, allowed the softened material to remain almost undisturbed.

In the case described on page 114 there was also softening of considerable extent, which may have been a factor in the occurrence of the hemorrhage. But apparently not so, the effusion simply breaking into this earlier focus as the direction of least resistance.

In Michel's case (*v.* p. 140, sub Spät-apoplexie) a large hemorrhage was attributed to softening of traumatic origin.

A case of abscess of right temporal lobe, with subsequent rupture of a vessel into this focus, is given by Dana (*Jrnl. N. and M. Dis.*, July, 1889, Case I.); this also broke through into the meninges.

Many cases, in corroboration, could be collected from other observers, but there is little occasion for doing so here.

The best evidence of this cause will be furnished by special cases that happen to be located, as in the two given, so near the surface as to break through without materially disturbing the previously softened material, and where, at the same time, death ensues so promptly that secondary changes have not taken place.

Though these two cases were meningeal (resp. ventricular), there is, *a priori*, no reason to suppose this form more frequently due to softening than the more common cases starting about the basal ganglia.

This etiology, due to previous softening, may be more common than appears. In most cases of brain-hemorrhage the torn-up and disintegrated tissues about the starting-point of the effusion make it impossible to say whether there was any preceding spot of necrosis or not. In doubt, it is classed under the more conservative head. A careful scrutiny with regard to this point, eventually with the help of an histological examination, can alone decide the frequency of this factor. From my experience it cannot be so exceedingly rare.

XVI.

CASES OF APOPLEXY FOLLOWING SOME TIME AFTER ACCIDENTS (DELAYED TRAUMATIC HEMIPLEGIA*).

It may be as well to begin with the facts that I have to offer, and discuss them briefly afterwards. The details are given not from any intrinsic interest but to establish the character of the cases.

CASE I.

Sarah C., eleven years old, seen in the summer of 1895. When fifteen months old she fell, with her mother, from the gang-plank of a steamer in landing at one of our inland lakes, but was rescued without injury so far as known. This occurred the last of August,—*i.e.*, in the warm season. Three weeks later she suffered a right hemiplegia (called "sudden" by the mother). This began of a Sunday morn-, ing. She first screamed ; then vomited (curdled milk only). A sister (then ten years old) says she immediately noticed that Sarah did not use her right side as well ; but it was not until evening that the hemiplegia was certified by a physician. During that first day she was sleepy and cried some, but was not strictly unconscious. It was some three weeks before she sat up again.

She began to talk when eight months old. After this attack she did not try to do so for three months. From

---

* Read in part before the "New York State Association of Railway Surgeons," at its sixth annual meeting, November 17, 1896.

that time on she spoke as readily as when she left off, and at present talks perfectly well.

At first, sensation was lost on the right side, as shown by burning her hand badly without appreciating it.

When she began to sit up there developed a twitching of the right side of the face. This part presently became perceptibly drawn, and remained so for a couple of years. No real paresis of the face now remains, though at times it seems to lag on the right.

Some five years ago she had the last of a series of peculiar attacks, evidently epileptic in character. In these she would start to run backward and then turn around. In the last one she fell backward down-stairs and sprained her wrist. Even now any sudden noise may start her to run forward.

She is a large-framed, well-nourished, bright-appearing girl. Weight, ninety pounds. No cardiac murmur. Right hand and arm are smaller, softer, and paler than the left. No real atrophy of muscles of right fore or upper arm, only the bones are smaller. This hand keeps in partial flexion, much like an obstetrical paralysis. Grip, l. 31, r. 0 (partly due to flexion, with no power in the extensors). Contact-sensation over right hand is very much reduced, though when perceived it is correctly located. Slight reduction of contact-sensation over right lower cheek border.

Methemiplegic movements on yawning and stretching, and of the right arm when squeezing with the left hand. Also on waking mornings she may put both hands over her head, a thing not possible voluntarily.

The walk shows a slight hitch and throw on the right. She sits in one uneasy twist if talking or at all excited, and is such a restless body that any thorough examination is difficult.

Pupils are equal, and each reacts well from all parts of retina (to ophthalmoscopic illumination). The hemiopic defect in the vision of each eye is fairly homonymous, as shown by the accompanying chart.

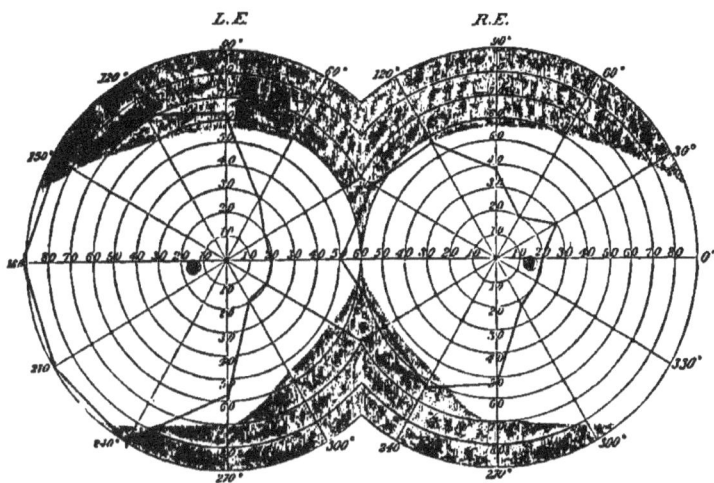

Outline of visual field in Case I.

Though taste and smell were asserted to be intact, the latter proved to be somewhat impaired on the left.

Hearing has long been supposed to be poorer on the left, but testing shows first one ear better, then the other.

Does fairly well in school ; is backward in mathematics if in anything. Whistles and loves music. "Sure to see the funny side of everything, and bound to have a good laugh." Again is rather sober.

CASE II.

Gentleman of forty-two years, referred to me by Dr. H. B. Delatour in February, 1896.

Has been troubled somewhat by asthma all his life. Otherwise was perfectly healthy and active until an accident seven years ago (in March, 1889). At that time he was thrown from a wagon, and chased the horse three hundred feet to catch it. Immediately on securing the animal he experienced a pain in the left occipital region. This kept up, but as he suffered no other inconvenience he still went about as usual. Just a week after the accident he was taken with the attack which disabled him. One morning, while waiting at a railroad station, he first noticed some trouble in speech,—could not say what he wanted to, neither could he write it. He got back home by train, recalls going into the house, but has no recollection further. In fact, the rest of that day he sat around and could say only " Don't know," or some such phrase. That night on retiring, and before he was in bed, he was heard to fall, and was found fully unconscious, breathing heavily (was even thought to be dead). His physician, Dr. J. W. Koontz, of Mount Jackson, Virginia, writes me that he found him suffering from a slight paralysis of the right side, with aphasia.—"I do not remember whether he suffered from nausea or not, but I rather think he did." "He remained unconscious for three weeks." When finally he came to he could not talk,—"a word or two at a time only." The face was also drawn to the left, as it is slightly even yet. After a month or so he was able to get about a little, dragging his right foot. It is claimed that ever since then he has been completely anæsthetic over left side of head, including mouth and tongue (cannot feel food on that side). But from the top of the neck down the anæsthesia is on the right side, and not quite so absolute.

During the hot weather last summer (1895) his left eye turned outward, the lid falling completely down. At present this is partly voluntary to cut off diplopia. He cannot open that eye as widely as the other, though the degree of ptosis varies. Previously there was none of this eye-trouble.

Formerly weighed two hundred and six pounds; about five years ago, one hundred and eighty ; now, one hundred and sixty. He has never weighed as much since the shock, but the total loss has been gradual. Very constipated since this trouble.

Heart-sounds clear. No bruit about head. Pulse varies on different days from 64 to 108 (the last following an attack of asthma).

Right hand very cool, a little puffy, at times trembly ; fingers nearly straight. Grip, r. 59, l. 88. No increase of wrist or arm reflexes on either side. Still writes exclusively with his right hand.

Pain-sense over right hand and thigh much impaired, somewhat also over calf. Touch (brush-contact, as also differentiation of two points) is very greatly reduced over the right side ; localization fair when once perceived.

While tests of cutaneous sensation over head give inconstant results, the following may pass as an average. Contact of fine brush against left half of face (including nose, chin, cheek, and fronto-temporal region) is not quite as easily detected as on the right. Esthesiometer over right facial region gave three centimetres ; over left, six centimetres ; localization in these areas is fair but not perfect. Pain-sense (pricking or electric brush) somewhat acuter over right side of head, though weaker even there. But temperature differences, apparently, were better perceived over the left side of head.

A very small spot on the cranium, an inch or so above and slightly back of exit of left occipital nerve, is decidedly tender to pressure and over-sensitive to the current. This is where he has had the pain since the accident, sometimes for months continuously, and, if anything, worse by day. Exit of occipitals not tender. One large, flat nuchal gland on the left.

In walking he uses a stick, and hitches or drags the right leg some,—literally "puts best foot forward," especially in going up-stairs. Cramps in hip and leg on right are common after sitting. There is, on the right, a slight knee-jerk from the tendon, but stronger from the patella. Left is variable, though usually weak.

Visual fields were as shown on the following chart. For

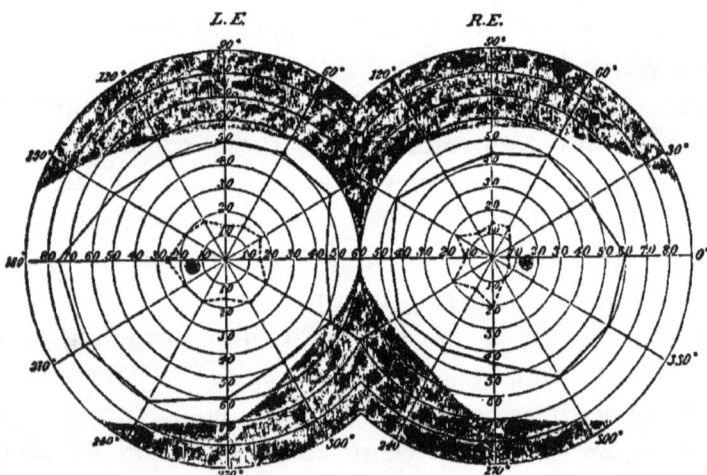

Visual field in Case II. Dotted line indicates limit for red.

the various colors perception was reduced correspondingly with that for red. This concentric limitation suggests that the visual deficiency here might be functional rather than definitely organic. Left pupil is a trifle wider than right. Left eye drops outward, and is poorly mobile,—upward to horizontal only, and inward but little beyond the middle line (doubtless paretic oculo-motor).

Watch heard on the right at three inches, on the left at three feet. Cannot hear slight sounds, or else fails to heed them.

Laughs or cries over-easily. Catches a joke quickly. Has much trouble in talking, the effort at times getting him into a general tremor. Often uses wrong word, and then tries to correct it, gesticulating frantically with his left hand. Has great difficulty in writing a letter, and always makes some mistakes. In writing from dictation often has to have it spelled. Can repeat after a person much better, though not perfectly. Has to hurry when he wants to urinate or do anything.

On September 12, 1896, Dr. Delatour trephined at the point of chief complaint. There appeared indications of a former fracture reaching forward and upward (slight depression in bone, and firm adhesion of pericranium and dura at the spot and in the direction indicated). The pia was free in all directions. Brain-surface grayish rather than pink, pulsating some.

Since this he has better control of muscles about the left eye, but otherwise there is little change.

In each of these cases the element of suits for damage was completely absent, and the evidence of organic mischief positive, so far as it can be without autopsy. They were cranial and not spinal cases. Aside from the brain-injury, each of these patients was still possessed of an excellent physique, still in the enjoyment of good health, and, though somewhat mobile of temperament, still cheerful as a rule. At the time of the accident neither had reached the favorite age for apoplexy.

It may be taken for granted that with such histories, relating to persons in youth or before any decline, no one will question the relation of cause and effect,—*i.e.*, that the accident induced the brain-trouble.

CASE III.

For the following case I am indebted to Dr. Philleo, of Brooklyn. The patient was a paver, over forty years of age, who had suffered a blow or fall on the head. He was brought to the hospital unconscious, but soon recovered. Discharged two and a half days later, apparently all right. He went back to his occupation and continued work for a whole week without any known or manifest symptoms. But eleven days after the accident he was brought in again and died promptly. The post-mortem examination revealed a fracture of the base that dated back to the time of the accident.

The following somewhat similar observations help to determine more definitely upon what pathological basis such cases depend.

Hilton ("Rest and Pain," New York, 1879, pp. 16, 17) says: "Some time since I was requested to see a gentleman in the country who, coming home from hunting, was thrown from his horse and got his foot entangled in the stirrup. In his fall he struck the back part of his head. After a time his horse was stopped; he disentangled his foot from the stirrup, and, expressing himself somewhat confused, mounted his horse again and rode several miles home. This gentleman occupied himself as usual during thirteen days, occasionally riding, sometimes walking, but more frequently driving about the country in the pursuit of his business and attending one of the county markets. He then became the patient of the surgeon who requested me to see him. At the time I saw him he was suffering from some indications of paralysis dependent on injury at the base of the skull or high up in the cervical region. This patient subsequently died, and upon examining his skull it was found that he had been the subject of a fracture of its base ; yet he pursued his ordinary avocations for thirteen days without the slightest evidence of any cerebral or brain lesion, complaining only of headache and some febrile condition."

Ewen, *Brit. Med. Jrnl.*, 1888, i. p. 899. A boy of ten years received a blow on the head. Not until sixty hours later did he complain of severe headache. Soon passed into coma with general relaxation. Death seventy-two hours after injury. Autopsy showed a thick clot, size of palm of hand, on the left side between dura and bone.

According also to Wiessmann, coma may be exceedingly delayed, one instance of eleven days being quoted.

Starr and McBurney, *Brain*, 1891. Man fell from a wagon. No loss of consciousness and no external wound. Several hours later he gradually became stuporous ; then unconscious for three days. Lasting aphasia, paralysis of right arm, and paresis of right leg. Partial right anæsthesia. Slight dementia. Trephining, with removal of a clot. Cure. This is attributed to hemorrhage from a vein of the pia.

My attention has been very kindly called by Dr. Townsend, of New York, to Scudder and Lund's paper (*Am. Jrnl. Med. Sc.*, April, 1895), giving data on the interval of consciousness between the occurrence of head-injuries and the development of coma from meningeal hemorrhage.

The longest period in any of their collected cases was two months (ten days longer before coma). This was in

Ceci's case, of the subdural form. In the extra-dural group, Ransohoff's case showed a free interval of eight days. The last writer (*Annals of Surgery*, 1890, vol. ii. p. 116) also discusses this point.

It appears that in about one-half of such cases there is some interval of consciousness after the injury.

Somewhat different is the recent case of E. Michel ("Ein Beitrag zur Frage von der sogenannten traumatischen Spätapoplexie," *Wiener klin. Wchr.*, 1896, No. 35, *v. Brln. kln. Wchr.*, 1897, i. p. 16).

"A man was injured by the falling of an iron bar, but showed no commotio cerebri. For a week he continued feeling comparatively well, except for some headache. Then severe brain-symptoms developed and he died. Autopsy showed : suffusion under the scalp on the right, but cranial bones intact ; hemorrhage between dura and pia, and into the pia on the right, more posteriorly ; blood-filled cavities in both occipital lobes, on the right to the outer side of and breaking into the ventricle ; ventricle full of blood ; numerous small hemorrhages in the vicinity of the blood-cavities and in the ependyma of the lateral ventricles. Apparently these small hemorrhages directly caused by the injury led to brain-softening, and in their further course to the fatal late apoplexy."

These various cases and citations indicate that meningeal bleeding (extra- or subdural) is the most common cause of delayed traumatic apoplexy. The reason for the striking delay in the development of symptoms is not so clear. In some cases there may have been oozing at the start or in the interval ; then came a more distinct vascular break. Again, it is an early or gradual accumulation, to which the brain is unable longer to accommodate itself.

There is a further group of cases resembling the above in the delayed development of paralysis, but without coma. Armstrong. *Jrnl. Am. Mcd. Assc.*, 1887, vol. i. p. 679. Negro of fifty-three years. Struck on left forehead by a brick. Scalp wound but no injury of bone. " Unconscious for a time." Then recovered, except for a roaring in his head, and wound healed. Right foot began to drag, just fifty days after accident, and developed into a hemiplegia. On trephining over left motor area and slightly opening dura, a quantity of "dark-brown blood" was evacuated. Recovery.

He quotes a case from Sylvestrini (1883) where temporary hemiplegia occurred two months after an accident, and full hemiplegia five months after. Trephining. Death.

Also a case from Grainger Stewart (*Brit. Med. Jrnl.*, 1887, i.) where headache began two weeks after accident, leading to hemiplegia. Trephining two months after. Death.

Fisher, of New York, has recorded an autopsy in which there was a large extra-dural hemorrhage that had existed for years, and yet caused no manifestations even at its origin.

Therapeutically we can draw the lesson that persons suffering from violence need care for some time. One indication is for quiet and sedatives. Avoid any excitement, exertion, or even mental stimulus. Depressants, especially of the blood-pressure, should be almost a routine treatment. Bromides, aconite, etc., are invaluable in warding off harm. There is also a strong indication for relief by trephining in these late cases, provided sufficient points for localization can be made out.

Those who follow practical medical work must continually be impressed by the closeness with which we have to correct our theories to assort with fact. Therefore the simple and honest relation of selected cases constitutes the basis of clinical knowledge. And such is my reason for offering you this report of cases, not in themselves especially novel, except that they represent, in one regard, a peculiar group, and one that *a priori* we should little expect to occur.

Furthermore, they are in a line that you, gentlemen of this society, must have unusually favorable opportunities of observing.

The various immediate results of accidents on the one hand, and the great group of late and indirect results (classed under railway spine or brain) on the other, are fully recognized. But well-marked cases of moderately delayed results ought to have interest not only in themselves, but also as showing conclusively that not all the evils of an accident develop in immediate sequence on the event.

P. S.—Mention might here be made of some experiments on the cadaver, made last summer with Dr. Mark Manley at the Kings County Hospital. These were to determine, if possible, the weak points in the dural arteries. Three times on two subjects pressure up to a hundred pounds to the square inch was tried, and yet without much success. In one case, where blows were directed to the parietal region during the injection, a slight effusion occurred in the upper parietal region. The injections were made at the base of the skull by introducing the cannula into the medi-dural through the slit-open external carotid. No better result was obtained in one trial where the calvarium had been removed from the opposite side.

XVII.

A CASE SUGGESTING MULTIPLE SCLEROSIS, BUT DUE TO CRANIAL ANEURISM.*

THIS is a case that has interested a number of medical men and been demonstated before several clinics.

The patient, C. A., of German parentage ; age, twenty-five years ; height, six feet one inch ; was admitted to the Kings County Hospital January 12, 1895.

At his occupation as a brass-finisher he has had to do much lifting of heavy weights,—really had often to hold and stem heavy objects against the polisher, thus prolonging the strain.

He has a noticeably dull and stupid or lubberly appearance ; his mother says he has always been so, and very slow to learn.

He dates back his trouble to four years ago. It began with the following symptoms. He first complained of a dull, continuous pain, which involved the whole right side of head. About one year subsequently he noticed a tremor of right hand, which increased in severity, compelling him to give up work. This was followed by inability to stand erect in one position for any length of time without liability of falling. At that time if he heard a noise while

---

* Reported by Dr. F. E. Lambert, late of the house-staff of the Kings County Hospital. Read before the Brooklyn Society for Neurology, February 28, 1895.

urinating it would excite him, causing the flow of urine to suddenly stop ; he would then be unable to urinate for several hours.

For the past year patient has been unable to walk without staggering, and says that if he heard any one behind him he would have to wait until they passed. About that time nystagmus, diplopia, and headache were troublesome. The tremor of right hand had gradually increased until he was unable to lift a cup of tea to the mouth without spilling its contents, the shaking increasing progressively as the hand approached the mouth.

His present symptoms include the following. His right hand shows great tremor of the intention type on every motion and effort, but is perfectly quiet while at rest. No tremor of left hand, which, however, in contrast to the right, is of a remarkable purple color, and usually cooler than the right. The color and appearance of right hand is normal. There is no motor paralysis of either hand, the relative power of the two being preserved. Arm and wrist reflexes normal and alike on the two sides.

On February 6 it is noted that for the past two nights the patient was awakened by pain in the little finger of the right hand ; it was dull in character and lasted about two hours. He also had pain in the adjoining finger and the corresponding finger of left hand.

It may be remarked, in passing, that patient has a congenital and symmetrical deformity of the little fingers.

When standing there is a continual fascicular and general trembling of whole right lower extremity (calf, thigh, and buttock), which entirely disappears when lying quietly, and does not involve the left leg, except by transmission of the vibration.

Both knee-jerks present; left the stronger. No ankle-clonus. When standing there is excessive incurve of lumbar spine (lordosis). His gait shows a peculiar hitch and faltering of the right side. No trophic disturbance noticed on the lower extremities.

There is a paresis of left lower facial; can scowl and close upper but not lower eyelid on that side. Draws mouth better to the right than to the left; noticeable also on laughing, and at times there is some twitching in the muscles of right cheek. This condition of the face, his mother says, has developed within the past two years. Noticeable atrophy of right half of tongue anteriorly. Tongue comes out straight, and palate hangs in the median line. Pharyngeal reflex seems absent. In speech there is some thickness, with mechanical hesitancy and catching at words.

The left pupil is larger, especially in twilight. Pupillary reaction is preserved on each side. Nystagmus of both eyes, more when looking upward or to either side, and some when looking down. It is a vertical nystagmus when looking upward, but lateral in all other positions. The right eye tends to turn a little out and upward. He also claims to see better with left eye. Diplopia most troublesome in distant vision. Ophthalmoscopic examinations show fairly normal conditions; right retina pale, disk distinct, and the arteries have the double contour. Veins full, and no pulsation observable. Condition of left retina similar. Examination disturbed by nystagmus.

General sensations were carefully examined by Dr. E. P. Hickok, assistant neurologist to department, who found no disturbance whatever as to contact, localization, or pain-senses. There is seborrhœa of scalp and somewhat of ears and eyebrows.

In attempting to make a diagnosis, at the time, several possibilities were considered. Against syphilis was a decidedly negative history, the absence of any other marks of it, and the futility of specific treatment.

The symptoms seemed hardly attributable to any form of brain-tumor.

In many respects, some form of multiple sclerosis was thought to offer a fair explanation (the tremor, though unilateral, nystagmus, speech-trouble, and various widely scattered symptoms), though not fully satisfactory. At a subsequent examination the following points were elicited. Pulsation of right side of neck is very much accentuated. This is distinctly visible below, in front of (temporal artery), and behind the right ear. Patient complains of a noise like a steam-engine in right ear. This proves to antedate all other symptoms, extending back six years. On the right side of neck, in the notch directly back of mastoid, on palpation a distinct purring sensation is felt with each beat, easily recognized as a full, strong aneurismal thrill. Mitral sounds normal ; aortic weak and a slight murmur with first beat. A continuous and very loud roar (venous hum) is heard over the right clavicle. The whirring noise from the mastoid can be distinctly heard over the entire cranium with each beat. Its character is almost as striking on diagonally opposite parts, over the malar prominence, or at any part solidly connected with the skull. Coughing or sneezing makes him quite dizzy. Hearing is defective, especially in right ear. He fails to readily discriminate sounds, and is quite oblivious to a low conversation. Can hardly distinguish the ticking of a watch, even in direct contact with right ear. Inspection of fauces shows fulness and pulsation on the right. Compression of the right common carotid completely stops the bruit, and almost completely arrests pulsation behind mastoid.

This evidence fully demonstrated the existence of an aneurism in some branch of the right carotid.

At first the external occipital appeared the most probable seat, as the palpable bruit is so far back; but the evident size of the dilatation, the fact that the internal artery is the one commonly involved, that tinnitus was a primary symptom, and that the souffle is so clearly heard at any point in the cranial bones, indicate the internal carotid as the vessel most probably affected. Or a fusiform and more extensive dilatation may be present. To cause all these symptoms the aneurism must not only exert a direct pressure,—as evidently on the outgoing hypoglossus to an extent that partly cuts the nerve off,—but also in some way involve adjacent intracranial structures. Whether this latter is an effect of the continual vibrations, or whether the enlargement pressed directly on the parts is fairly answered by the later course of the trouble. It was, at any rate, clear that some effort should be made to cure the aneurism. It was proposed to the patient to tie one vessel first, and if later this proved insufficient, the other could be treated in like manner.

Dr. A. T. Bristow kindly saw the patient, coincided in the indications, and on February 21 ligated the right common carotid. The patient recovered somewhat slowly but excellently from the operation, and made uninterrupted progress for a time. By February 24 several of the most prominent symptoms had almost entirely disappeared, among them being the tremor of right hand, headache, purple color of left hand, the ear-noises, as also the objective bruit and local fulness on palpation.

Two weeks after the operation his condition was still better. The tremor of hand appeared only on prolonged extension, and then even was but slight. Ordinarily speaking, there was no tremor; he could put right hand to mouth without a quiver. From the absence of ear-distraction he seemed much brighter. Heard watch at two feet (right). Nystagmus less. Power in the two hands still in proportion (r. 69, l. 66). The state of the lower extremity could not yet be certainly determined, as he had been kept quiet in bed and under moderate doses of gelsemium, with a view to favoring a maximum shrinkage of the aneurismal sac.

March 20, 1895. Some local pulsation, especially under right ear, though scarcely as much as on left. The thrill is audible behind right ear; the notch there is even more palpable.

Cough disturbs his head, making, especially on left side of head, "a dragging feeling," whatever that may mean. His head, when sitting quietly, vibrates or oscillates back and forth quite noticeably with each pulsation. The left hand is again somewhat purple and cooler than the right. The tremor of right hand has increased again a trifle, though still but slight. He can walk alone, though the right leg is the poorer, at least there is some twist and hitch in gait. More headache; worse when lying down; after fifteen or twenty minutes such a dizzy ache he can hardly sleep; still, to-day all his symptoms are, he says, mending again.

As to his prospects for the future, all depends on a recurrence of the aneurism. There is the possibility that a quiet life or eventually further ligations may control it. In any event, the case remains one of great clinical interest.

XVIII.

APOPLEXIES OF THE BRAIN. THE IMPORTANCE OF EARLY
TREATMENT BASED ON THE DIFFERENTIAL DIAGNOSIS
OF THE SEVERAL FORMS (HEMORRHAGE, EMBOLISM,
THROMBOSIS, PSEUDO-SEIZURES).*

PERHAPS evolution has not kept pace with the augmented
demands on our brain-vessels. At least there is an im-
pression that troubles of this kind are more prevalent than
in primitive times. Be that as it may, the subject of their
medical care is well worth attention.

The causes and prophylaxis of apoplexy are, to some
extent, understood ; but there seems to be a lack of any
promising or systematic line of treatment when actual
trouble begins. We all know the uselessness of incisive
measures in cases of this class after the condition has become fully established. As it is at this stage that the spe-
cialist is usually called in, it is the more important that the
proper course to adopt at the beginning—the only time
when there is hope of our being of great service—should
be understood by the profession as generally as possible.
For in a considerable proportion of cases invaluable help can
be rendered if the physician first called is familiar with the
requirements. I know full well how often we are too late,
or at best unable to accomplish much, and yet in very
many cases we can, if duly alert, be of service ; and even

---

* Read, in part, before " The Medical Club," Brooklyn, June 24, 1895.

though the full evil be accomplished before our arrival, it is safer to proceed on the basis that it is not so.

Many say, What is the use, the patient is sure soon to have a relapse? But this is not so certain ; the person may still be good for years of activity. And while the average of expectation in such an individual may be short, it should be remembered that one year at this usually mature time of life is often of more account to the dependent family than a decade of youth. In any case, however, our duty is beyond question.

The plan of treatment here proposed is, for each type, one of strict rationalism, and depends on simple mechanical principles. The application of these may not be new in any regard ; and yet the errors met in practice, and, still more, the wild and useless recommendations that we so often see advocated in print, suggest that some one ought to make a systematic presentation of what can be done and how to do it. Many of our therapeutic attempts are based on the blind action of remedies or drugs that, even if active, may or may not accomplish some indirect result that we desire. Here we have an important field in which we can work on clear lines, for a definite purpose, and with controllable but positive means.

It is proposed to take up specifically but the four classes of cases. What I have to say is based on my own observations, and every point I believe I have had opportunity to verify in practice. One unfortunate fact often limits the exactness of our knowledge in these matters, and that is the difficulty of getting autopsies.

DIAGNOSIS.

The first matter in any given case is an exact differential diagnosis between the conditions under consideration.

Upon this depends all our hope of usefulness, since they call, in part, for directly opposite lines of treatment. Unfortunately, the means of distinguishing, especially in such emergency cases, are inadequate. I can mention but a few,—for the most part but little recognized in the books, and some of which deserve a more careful consideration ; even though "adventitious" symptoms, they are of the highest importance,—and emphasize the necessity of good medical judgment. To know our patients, their past histories, and any chronic disorders from which they may be suffering, is more than half the battle.

With us hemorrhage seems to be the most frequent form, although from studies elsewhere this may be more apparent than real.

Its occurrence under forty years of age has been supposed to indicate embolism, and over forty, hemorrhage. Yet there are too many exceptions to allow much value to any such age-rule. Gowers ("Clinical Lectures," 1895, p. 57) says, " These two [embolism and thrombosis from syphilitic disease, as causes of hemiplegia] embrace certainly ninety-five per cent. of the cases of sudden onset in early adult life."

Renal disease with its arterial changes may cause hemorrhage, often false attacks of uræmic nature, less often thrombosis, but not of itself ever embolism.

It is doubtful if an excess of adipose, either general or especially about the neck, has any relation to the rupture of encranial vessels,—the sparest physique is no guarantee of immunity. On the contrary, I have so often seen it occur in frail females (emaciation not due to nephritis) that there must be some very opposite factor in play. Dr. Matthews, of Brooklyn, suggested, apropos of such a case,

an old principle as affording a reasonable explanation,—
the ex-vacuo theory. The brain-vessels in such a person
lack the necessary support that they have in a well-nourished individual, and so in time give way. This view is
borne out in my experience by the fact that in such a
person the hemorrhage when once started has always been
a very large one (no counter-pressure to check the outflow).
The principle may help us to understand such cases, though
it affords no material assistance in making a differential
diagnosis.

It has been suggested that the onset on rising in the
morning may be of diagnostic value. Its occurrence at
this time is not very rare, though it is not always possible
to ascertain definitely whether or not it existed before first
rising. At the instant of assuming the upright position
there is a sudden letting-down of the brain-current, sufficient in a weak person to produce symptoms of fainting.
To that extent thrombosis would be favored. But this
stage is too temporary by itself to cause that result, and
is followed by an increase in the heart's action and a
heightening of the blood-pressure. An embolus might be
set going or, more likely, a vessel ruptured.

If, however, the condition was found before rising, the
probability would be thrombosis or hemorrhage,—embolism
not impossible, but only unlikely.

In persons who have had spontaneous hemorrhages elsewhere, as under the conjunctiva, there is a natural inclination to make a diagnosis of like cerebral effusion. But I
have seen this very occurrence followed soon after by
evident cerebral thrombosis with continued inclination to
recur.

Several medical friends have related to me cases in their

practice where the onset of an apoplexy was at the time of coitus.* These few cases seem always to have been in the male ; but like attacks in the female, and apparently of cerebral origin, are now and then heard of. It is clear that the greatly heightened vascular tension during this act would prevent any thrombosis at the time. An embolus might be swept off, but the probabilities are strongly in favor of hemorrhage in such an event.

Straining at stool is an occasional cause. This ought likewise not to favor embolism. It might permit thrombosis, though its special tendency would be towards vascular tearing and hemorrhage.

The occurrence of vomiting is common, and strongly suggestive of hemorrhage, but not of embolism or thrombosis. Nausea, of course, may attend nephritis, and dizziness, faintness, etc., occur in thrombosis ; but real vomiting, aside from uræmia (the person being in a prone position), argues in a suspicious case for hemorrhage. Of course, any existing kidney-trouble augments both hemorrhage and nausea. In fact, vomiting is one of the most important and decisive symptoms. This applies to the increasing period of the hemorrhage. Where the latter is at all voluminous, in almost any part of the brain, we get vomiting, severe and often somewhat prolonged. Its occurrence depends (aside from personal idiosyncrasy) upon the volume of the effusion, still more upon the speed with which it is poured out, and to some extent also upon its location. In the slower or ingravescent forms, even though they finally reach a large size, there is much less tendency to emesis.

---

* An occurrence long since discussed by Bertini, *Gior. d. Soc. Med.-chir. di Torino*, 1843, vol. xvi. pp. 67–69.

It is only where we find other evidence of an apoplectic seizure that this symptom is of value, and then chiefly in differentiating the nature of the brain-process.

Nearly always some other plausible explanation of the vomiting is proffered. The person has just eaten over-heartily, or been lying in a cramped position, or had a hypodermic, or taken medicine that upset the stomach, or been suffering from gastric catarrh. The regularity and persistency with which this manifestation in these cases is misinterpreted is almost pathognomonic.

When the condition develops during sleep the probabilities are against embolism. It may be a hemorrhage, while it is a favorite time for thrombosis, thanks to the ebb in circulation.

A history of past rheumatism, especially the presence of a heart-murmur, and sometimes a knowledge of previous vascular plugging (immaterial in what part of the body), speak for embolism. Says Gowers, *l. c.*, p. 55, "To justify a diagnosis of embolism you must find a source,—that is, practically you must find valvular disease of the heart ; or, if the attack occurred some months ago, you must have a history of some malady, not long before the onset, known to cause endocarditis." This ignores cases due to the breaking down of atheromatous patches, oftener transient.

Usually embolic symptoms develop suddenly and are soon complete, this giving a very useful diagnostic help, though they *may* deepen for hours after the onset.

Gowers, *l. c.*, p. 58, "Loss of consciousness at the onset is chiefly important when the distinction has to be made between hemorrhage and softening.' In the latter it is more often absent than present. . . . The only help it gives is that it is rather more often absent in thrombosis than in embolism, because the latter is more violently sudden." Embolism is somewhat less liable to cause coma ; at any rate, the deep stertorous condition. I have elsewhere shown (*Medical News*, February 18, 1888) that embolism limited to the pallium (cortex and centrum ovale) is *not* attended by coma. Slowly developing or late loss of consciousness speaks somewhat against embolism and suggests a vast hemorrhage or progressing thrombosis, resp., of course, inflammation.

Previous headaches, apparently in relation to the present trouble, count against embolism.

Yawning, and especially sighing, at times in respiration are very frequent and noticeable symptoms in hemorrhage, and also in thrombosis and its precedent conditions. There is a slight parallelism between this and the vomiting. These manifestations are often more marked if the person sits up. But unfortunately they have but a limited value, as the embolic subject often has a heart so damaged that the same evidence of brain-anæmia will be presented.

Excessively warm weather, a rapid rise in the atmospheric temperature, and very likely marked fall of the barometric pressure greatly favor the occurrence of thrombosis, while opposed to hemorrhage.

That the heated term through its general debilitating action favored sinus-thrombosis in children has long been known. My observations indicate that such meteorological conditions also greatly favor arterial thrombosis in adults, though in a different manner. The debilitating influence may, of course, be a part factor. There is a more important one, so far as the arteries are concerned, in the dilatation of the peripheral circulation with consequent drawing away from the brain, and coincident with this the general enervating effect of a heated atmosphere.

Prolonged and wavering prodromata, especially if diffuse or scattering and not focal, past syphilis, debility, and exhaustion also suggest thrombosis. The unilateral type of paræsthesiæ, especially where not continuous and coming on in an elderly person, possibly accompanied by some dizziness and slight nausea, is strongly suggestive of threatening thrombosis.

It was long supposed that these peculiar tinglings, etc. (pallor, headache, dizziness, fulness in the head, visual obscuration, nausea, numbness of one side), pointed to impending hemorrhage. Of late, owing to inability to account for such premonitions, there has been a disinclination to recognize any connection of the kind. In view of the evidence of a vaso-motor influence, as given in the chapter on symmetrical brain-hemorrhages, it is probable that local paralysis of vessels with sufficient dilatation to irritate adjacent tracts may precede the actual rupture. This, however, is usually more continuous, and ends within a few days in a frank attack of apoplexy. If before senility it is also more suggestive of threatening rupture.

"Atheroma is a disease of the old, even more emphatically than is hemorrhage, for in extreme old age it becomes the more common lesion of the two." Gowers, *l. c.*, p. 57.

The physiologically recurring waves of vessel-contraction and diurnal or other periods of fall in pressure, added to the pathological narrowing of the vessel (where there is danger of thrombosis), may evidently for a time limit the nourishment in the respective area sufficiently to injure its function without actually causing necrosis. The tissues are still supplied with enough to keep them alive, and as soon as

the flow again increases these resume their functions.   Presently, however, if relief is not obtained, the matter goes too
far and irreparable softening ensues.

Gowers, *l. c.*, p. 56, "Thrombosis has two causes.   It is
a clotting of the blood, and it may be due only to a strong
tendency of the blood to clot.   This, however, is rare.   It
occurs in the old and gouty ; it occurs in the subjects of
cancer ; it occurs in states of profound general weakness ;
and it occurs especially soon after childbirth, when the
vessels of the uterus have to be closed by clot. . . . The
second cause of thrombosis to which we are reduced is
disease of the artery at the spot, disease which induces
formation of the clot."

Thrombosis is largely secondary to alterations in the
coats of the vessels.   So the syphilitic form is hardly a
simple deposit from the blood.   It may be essentially a
blocking by thickening of the arterial well (*in specic* of the
intima).   But clinically, and to some extent practically, it is
the same thing.   There may be distinguishing marks, and,
of course, a knowledge of antecedent specific trouble is
important.   In my experience, despite some authorities,
the process tends to involve many vessels or branches
either at the same time or in succession.   Its purely passive phenomena may also irregularly rise and fall for some
time, as just pointed out,—one day or part of a day present,
then abating and recurring.   One picture of this kind resembles the condition termed astasia-abasia.   The patient,
for instance, cannot read long without blurring or loss of
concentration (dyslexia) ; cannot talk without presently getting a word wrong, or, more often, failing to command the
language desired.   In attempting to write, the head soon
rebels and little errors creep in ; long calculation or accus-

tomed continuous thinking is impossible, and much muscular exertion soon tires. And yet there is no paralysis nor real paresis, nor falling out of any function. *The centres act normally for a brief period, then play out.** This may apply to large areas or almost the whole brain, again is more one-sided or even further limited. Occasionally in persons of some intellectuality it is quite possible to locate the phenomena in the field of one or more arteries, preferably the sylvian or its branches. In this specific form, which may occur at almost any period of life, there may, or oftener may not, be much headache; if especially nocturnal, so much the more in evidence. In other forms of trouble here considered preceding headache is not rare.

The fact that compression of the carotids may aggravate existing symptoms, and even bring on slight convulsions in persons suffering from arterio-sclerosis or other impairment of the brain-circulation (Naunyn and others), suggests it as an expedient in the diagnosis of thrombosis. But as it must tend to affect disadvantageously such a patient's cerebral condition, and possibly involve injury to the carotids, it should be resorted to only with great care.

There are two other classes of cases in which hemiplegia results where it is desirable to have more exact knowledge, —viz., those following (1) infectious diseases; (2) accidents.

Applying the facts brought together by J. J. Thomas ("Diphtheritic Hemiplegia," *Am. Jrnl. Med. Sci.*, April, 1896), we must conclude that those resulting from infections may be either hemorrhagic, embolic, or thrombotic.

---

* This is quite distinct from the prolonged, dazed, stuporous condition sometimes seen in younger females with active syphilis.

The other form, that supervening some time after accidents, is considered in a special chapter.

Assuming, now, that the diagnosis is made, we can take up the treatment of each form.

I. HEMORRHAGE OF THE BRAIN.

In these cases there is a wide range as to location, size, and tendency to spontaneous cessation. Some are promptly fatal, meningeal and ventricular forms being usually of this kind. Nearly always, however, as pointed out by Liddell, the effusion progresses for some time. In numerous cases the ingravescent type is approached, and just to that extent there is time in which we can act. Even if the outflow has already stopped, it is right to make this doubly sure, and head off any early recurrence.

Our efforts should be directed to a lowering of the arterial pressure, and to a deviation of the blood-current to other parts, —i.e., *in general to a reduction of the supply to the brain.*

There are several available and trusty methods of accomplishing this,—

(1) Position of the Patient. Some have recommended lying with the head low, while a New York colleague has advocated the erect posture, and Heidenhain (1890) the attitude of sitting. *The main essential is a sufficiently prone attitude to insure a complete relaxing of all the muscles,* since we know that all muscular effort tends to increase the arterial tension. And independent of the play of the muscles, the blood-pressure is, I believe, known to be greater in the erect posture. Granted, then, the reclining position, shall the head be dropped or kept moderately elevated? A little observation of the ways of mankind suffices to furnish an answer. Persons suffering from simple

anæmia and exhaustion naturally sleep with the head low, this evidently favoring the brain-supply. And every surgeon knows that to resuscitate a patient the first thing is to lower the head. On the other hand, persons with an overactive brain-circulation sleep with the head high, sometimes lowering it towards morning as the pressure subsides (*v.* "The Morning Headache of Exhaustion," *Brkn. Med. Jrnl.*, 1891, p. 40). In heart-lesions also, doubtless to modify the shock of each beat and to pass the blood from chest and head to dependent parts, the sufferer courts a higher elevation of the head. These facts are so clear and convincing as to settle the question of attitude,—unless, of course, to meet the exigencies of some unusual circumstance.

In conclusion, then, the favorite position for a patient with progressive cerebral hemorrhage should be with the body sufficiently reclining to be fully relaxed and the head considerably elevated.

Other matters of posture may need attention. The vomiting in such a case appears to be eased by turning the person on the right side ; the thought being to thus favor the natural discharge of the stomach into the intestine. Certainly the vomiting act in itself must greatly tend to increase the cerebral outflow. But Robert L. Bowles advocates turning the patient over on the paralyzed side to ease stertor.

(2) Vaso-drugs. The proper use of these remedies is probably the most valuable single resource we have. Of course, ergot is generally discarded,—no one ever really found out whether it did harm or good. In the cardiovascular depressants—gelsemium, veratrium, aconite, or possibly pilocarpine—we have a means powerful enough to suit any one, effective and yet ordinarily safe. My own

preference is for gelsemium, very likely because of its greater general paralyzing action. This ought, doubtless, for its quickest effect, to be used hypodermically, though it acts promptly by the mouth. The fluid extract can be started in adults with an initial dose of two to five drops and followed by drop-doses at intervals dependent on the closeness with which the case can be watched. It should be pushed until its physiological action is manifest, whether little or much is required. For the time paralyze your patient. There may be contra-indications as regards the use of these drugs, but I have rarely had occasion to heed them in such cases.

When medication on this line has to be continued for any length of time, however, it may be necessary to change, especially from full doses of gelsemium. Then the others become useful. Veratrium is next in order ; and both because of the more general familiarity of the profession with this drug, and of our knowledge of its safety from the ample experience of its use in puerperal eclampsia, it will with most practitioners prove the most acceptable remedy right from the start.

It is usually advisable to keep up some influence of this kind from a couple of days to a week at least.

Be careful, on the contrary, to avoid all stimulants, vascular tonics, morphine (resp. any opiate of this class), and, for the time, strychnine. Digitalis I have repeatedly known to bring on a recurrence a few days after the primary attack. The use of nitroglycerin in the developing stage of brain-hemorrhage almost certainly does harm, and should, for this particular purpose, be abandoned.

The possibility of increasing the coagulability of the blood by internal drugs is as yet visionary.

11

(3) Constriction of the Extremities. This is a very promptly acting but temporary expedient with many limitations. Care must be had that the vessels are not so brittle as to be injured by the compression, that just sufficient force is used to more or less shut off the veins without affecting the arteries (if too much we but strangle the extremity, if too little we fail of our purpose), that the respective extremities do not become too cold, and, finally, that the constriction be eased up very gradually lest the sudden influx into the general circulation again start up the very trouble we are seeking to control. Warm bottles at the extremities and gentle frictions are of themselves useful in drawing blood to the parts, and are doubly so when constriction is used.

The recently vaunted compression of the carotids is a doubtful therapeutic measure (its possibilities for diagnostic purposes have already been considered), as the vessels in these patients are often easily injured, a steady control of the current for any length of time is rarely possible, and the frequent jets that do get by the compressor's fingers must wonderfully tend to displace any occluding clot at the point of rupture. Ligature of a carotid seems a still more crazy and quite unnecessary procedure.

Ice to the head is a very popular plan, but also of very uncertain value. Probably, if used at all for the purpose, the ice might far better be applied over the carotids in the neck.

(4) Depletion of Body-fluids. Formerly this was the main treatment, and practised in the form of venesection. Many still think highly of this for some cases. The most common and still accepted method is by purgatives, as a drop of croton oil on the tongue. Or a glycerin enema may be given.

In cases of threatening rather than developing hemorrhage of the brain, laxatives are most important. Fer-
mentation, clogging, etc., of the bowels seem at times an
immediate cause, and then calomel is particularly in place.

Pilocarpine might be admirable, since it acts both as a
depressant and as a fluid-depletor, but for certain risks, as
of pulmonary œdema.

It will perhaps not be amiss, in passing, to contrast with
the foregoing our limited resources in the second stage of
apoplexy. For convenience we can distinguish three different stages,—

1st. That of onset and development, already considered.

2d. That of reaction (or subacute).

3d. The chronic, remaining after all active processes have
run their course (unless the degeneration of implicated
paths).

In the second stage there is still some shock, an actual
destruction of brain-tissue, a compression of adjacent tracts
by the volume of the extravasation, and an inflammatory
reaction of immediately surrounding parts. It is largely
the development of this last that constitutes the final factor
in so many cases ending fatally in from two to ten days.
Moreover, where life is retained the neighboring structures
are by this reaction, œdema, etc., still further jeopardized,
and the possible extent of eventual recovery is materially
reduced.

It might be thought that there would be more hope of
late improvement after hemorrhage than after infarction.
Yet experience hardly bears this out, the reason therefor
probably being the greater reaction surrounding a hemorrhage.

We have little to offset this. Counter-irritation can

hardly act that deeply. Iodides to favor quick absorption of clot, and brucia or its congeners to support the viability of endangered fibres, is about all. Trephining, with evulsion of clots, would be in order, though so rarely feasible. Of course, we can also do something towards warding off a recurrence. Negatively, the use of digitalis in a patient who has once suffered from brain-hemorrhage is ever after a risky matter.

II. EMBOLISM OF THE BRAIN.

The treatment of this condition is in nearly every respect the direct opposite of that for hemorrhage.* Three ways of relief suggest themselves.

a. The first is by the development of a collateral circulation. But, as is well known, certain portions of the brain supplied with terminal vessels are excluded from such possibility ; and even the vessels of the other parts have so limited connections as to preclude full compensation where an artery of much size is stopped. The means favoring a development of collaterals are the same as those described below (*sub c*).

b. Another is by breaking up the embolus. In practice, however, we cannot expect in any manner to accelerate this, except so far as it may be favored by increased pressure and the act of tumbling the plug along. Something in this line may be more certainly accomplished where the blockage is due to soft atheromatous material.

c. The final and really available way is to force the embolus as far along into some peripheral vessel as possible. Any advance is a great gain. An inch may reduce the area jeopardized to but a fraction of its original extent,—

---

* Bastian (1890) partly appreciates this when he notes that hemorrhage requires directly opposite methods of treatment from embolism and thrombosis.

and this means much more to the patient than such a ratio indicates. Then there is better chance of the collateral circulation sufficing. Hence the general plan is to hoist the flood-gates and turn on pressure.

1. Sometimes the heart is beating violently, and we fear lest another plug be torn off. Or the patient may not be in good trim for being up ; or many times the heart is too enfeebled to properly overcome gravity. So that the wisest and safest rule is to place the head very low, even letting it be dependent.

2. Here the nitrites are directly indicated, the quickly acting nitroglycerin or nitrite of amyl being best. Then come alcoholics in doses to stimulate. Next free libations of hot drinks that may rapidly be taken up by the circulation. Probably hot cloths along the carotids in the neck would be useful, as dilating the supply-tubes of the respective area.

Avoid scrupulously all depressants, depletors, and such vascular constrictors as ergot and digitalis. Strophanthus may be admissible.

Abdominal bandaging à la Leonard Hill (*Proc. Roy. Soc., v. N. Y. Med. Jrnl.,* 1895, i. pp. 349, 350), though employed by him for other conditions, would be worth using here. And even an Esmarch to one or more extremities would be quite in order.

For embolism, then, favorable position of head and body, dilatation of brain-vessels, heightening of blood-pressure where safe, increase of body-fluids.

III. THROMBOSIS.

This is a far more complicated subject, and the treatment partakes much more of a prophylactic nature. The trouble is usually of slower development and needs be met with less vigor but more persistence. It is quite as serious as the previous troubles, much more varied in nature, and requires greater skill in adaptation of means to an end. There is one serious danger in the measures for relief. We are dealing with diseased vessels, their walls being often much weakened. There is no such disturbing fear in embolism, for there the vessels are presumably healthy, nor in hemorrhage, for there our efforts at relief involve no strain on the vessels. Just as I have seen an œsophageal stricture cause a rupture of its adjacent wall, so I always fear in treating cerebral thrombosis lest the therapeutic efforts bring on an equally objectionable hemorrhage.

Hemorrhage usually and embolism always is arterial, while thrombosis may affect veins or sinuses as well as arteries. The sinus form is a somewhat special matter, following either neighboring septic trouble or else exhaustion and debility, notably in children, while thrombosis of cerebral veins can hardly be distinguished as an entity by itself. In the arterial form of adults we know of three principal causes,—arterio-fibrosis in nephritics, atheroma, and the end-arteritis of syphilis. When from either of these causes we find signs of danger impending or trouble already present, the first or immediate line of treatment is analogous to that in embolism, though there is less need of increasing the body-fluids. The vessels must be dilated to allow the blood to pass, and the pressure should be increased to get it through. Here, again, the nitrites are as yet the sheet-anchor, sometimes reënforced by strophanthus and strychnine. But there is a choice. The nitrite of sodium or even of potassium is the best, since its action is more

prolonged than that of the amyl or glycerin com-
pounds.*

Avoid digitalis and everything causing arterial contraction. As soon as immediate relief is secured we must take
some course for more lasting benefit.

1st. In kidney-trouble this may not be possible, our
treatment there remaining symptomatic.

2d. In atheroma the French commend small long-con-
tinued doses of iodide of potassium. For one reason or
another (slow action, the occurrence of iodism, etc.) it has
rarely given much satisfaction in my experience.

But there are several useful lines of treatment. The
nitrites should be accompanied or followed by brucia or its
allies in stout doses (one-twentieth to one-thirty-second
of a grain), and persisted in for months with more or less
regularity according to immediate needs at any time.

Another useful line of remedies depends upon the fact
that most of these old patients are rheumatic, gouty, or suf-
ferers from what may be termed senile lithæmia. Physical
inactivity plays a part. The waste and refuse products of
the system are not eliminated with due promptness and
aggravate the atheromatous processes. Here alkalies and
antilithic remedies have to be employed. One of the most
important aids is furnished by certain of the sulphur waters.
If it is possible for the patient to visit the springs, so much
the better ; otherwise the water may be employed at home.

---

* Bradbury, in a recent Bradshaw Lecture on some new vaso-dilators (*Lancet,* 1895, vol. ii. pp. 1205–1213), brings experimental proof of the avail-
ability of erythrol tetra-nitrate and mannitol nitrate. In doses of a grain or
even more (given either in solid form or dissolved in alcohol) the effect begins
in half an hour and lasts several hours. These are non-poisonous and do not
cumulatively lose their action like nitroglycerin.

Sharon, Massena, or other waters of this class can be had in bottles and used anywhere. The water should be taken up to a half-pint before breakfast and supper for periods of a month or more at a time. After an interval the course may need to be repeated. The good the patient experiences from these waters is often not limited to any effect on the brain-arteries, but includes a favorable action on many other functions of the body.

This use of these waters seems to be little known, but I can commend it as a valuable addition to our means.

In syphilis the whole power of our therapeutic resources should be forthwith brought to bear, and continued until long after all symptoms are gone or all hope of relief abandoned. It should be borne in mind that often the so-called specifics for syphilis will develop this desired local action only after the vessels have been dilated. When they are almost closed, it is evident that little blood, and consequently little of the medicament, can reach the imperilled point. It is necessary, if possible, to open the vessel-path, and, while keeping the way open, follow up with the more direct specifics.

This field for the use of vaso-dilators has not been properly, if at all, recognized. In my experience their value is very great, and their effect strikingly satisfactory to patient and physician. Once we have a correct diagnosis, if destruction has not already taken place, the certainty of at least temporary relief is as great as in any trouble about which we are consulted.

As syphilis has such a wide-spread tendency to cause arterial interference, the same principle is applicable in many of its late forms. To what extent it will prove useful in securing more effect of the specifics when other parts of the body are involved may be left to those working in those lines to decide. One of my colleagues, Dr. Winfield, has adopted it in many of these old cases, and believes it to be a success. We all know that at times an undoubted syphilitic process fails to respond well to treatment. Some of these cases can be reached by this plan, and very many by a less amount of specifics than otherwise.*

IV. PSEUDO-APOPLECTIC SEIZURES.

(IN PART THE APOPLEXIA NERVOSA AND PARAPOPLEXY OF OLDER WRITERS.)

UNDER this heading might be included a great variety of conditions due to fainting, hysteria, congestive chills, toxæmias, as gout, disseminated sclerosis, cerebral softening of unknown origin, etc. But I refer to a type best illustrated by the paralytic and convulsive attacks that not rarely occur in the early course of paresis. Clinically and practically there is quite a parallelism between these and

---

* Recently Petrone, of Naples, induced by certain chemical considerations, made a trial of the nitrite in syphilis ("Sull 'uso dei nitriti nella cura delle Malattie infettive," *Riforma Medica*, 1895. Agosto. Abstr. in *Giornale Italiano delle Malattie Veneree e della Pelle*, September, 1895). One case was of combined paludism and syphilis. Initial dose of five to ten centigrammes, increased to a maximum of half a gramme daily. This was given subcutaneously in solutions of two to three per cent.,—five per cent. may be painful. Treatment lasted thirty days. Second case was a woman of twenty-two years, with hereditary syphilis. Treatment as in preceding case for twenty-six days. Complete cure. Sprecher, of Turin, *ibid.* (*Giornale Italiano*, 1896, pp. 453–456), found in twelve cases that it only relieved osteocopic pains, and even that much with uncertainty, and often discomfort.

But these observers used it as a remedy in itself for the disease, and hence for a very different purpose. The method employed by me is first for temporary safety, and then more widely as a means by which to get better results from routine specifics. For this purpose the hypodermic use is unsuited ; prolonged action without untoward effects is that here desired.

certain manifestations of chronic alcoholism. Their correct recognition may require our finest diagnostic skill, and yet is usually possible and even certain, medically speaking.

Such paralyses may be found in the morning, yet without adequate shock; or come on during waking hours without much general disturbance, though usually attended by many distinguishing symptoms. They are, as a rule, of brief duration, beginning to improve in a day or two. Allied to these, and frequently associated with them, are the more common epileptiform convulsions, not rarely very severe in character.

The key to one line of rational and relatively successful treatment here is given by certain pathological findings. In old alcoholics we expect the wet brain, with the effused fluid under decided pressure. It has also long been known that there was an excess of fluid about the brains of paretics. Writers call this *ex vacuo*. Nevertheless the fluid many times spurts out on incising the dura. If pressure still persisted post-mortem, how much greater must it have been during life. In fact, this is conclusive proof that the accumulation is *not* passive to fill up any vacuum; and the argument must hold even for cases where we have less evidence of pressure, despite the fact that many of the authorities conclude otherwise.

Again, the good that some operators have seen follow trephining in dements argues against the vacuum view.

Perhaps the most accepted teaching as to the immediate causation of these seizures is that they depend on local cerebral œdemas or fluxions. This is in harmony with the above. Hence we have a definite basis for action.

It will not do to draw the blood away from the head, as a compression-anæmia already exists, and is presumably the very cause of the attacks. We must get the fluid away, stimulate its absorption, and support the blood-pressure. Diuretics, like iodide of potash, cardiac stimulants, like strophanthus, and counter-irritation, as by small fly-blisters over the scalp and back of the mastoids, are of grand service. Bromides are useless, even harmful, though so often prescribed. Spinal puncture (suggested for paresis by the writer in 1894) is theoretically indicated, though in my experience so inadequate as to be almost useless. Recently Babcock (*State Hospital's Bulletin*, July, 1896), has reported some benefit from this procedure in progressive dementia ; though J. Turner (*Brit. Med. Jrnl.*, 1896, vol. i. p. 1084) observed practically no amelioration in fourteen cases.

Trephining with incision of the dura is rational, but any operation requiring the administration of an anæsthetic is in that way decidedly objectionable.

What we need here, as in several other troubles, is some plan for increasing the normal absorption of the fluid, some improved drainage from the subarachnoid meshes back into the general lymphatics.

It may not be amiss. in closing to call attention to the need of common sense in applying any remedy. The special conditions in some concrete case may warrant us in directly contravening the best of rules.

Finally, a given set of measures should not be condemned because, unhappily, often inadequate to the requirements If they are unquestionably rational we should use them for all they are worth, and at the same time hunt for further help.

The main original purpose of this paper was to show how widely the therapeutic indications differed in these classes of cases.

PLATE I.

FIG. 1.

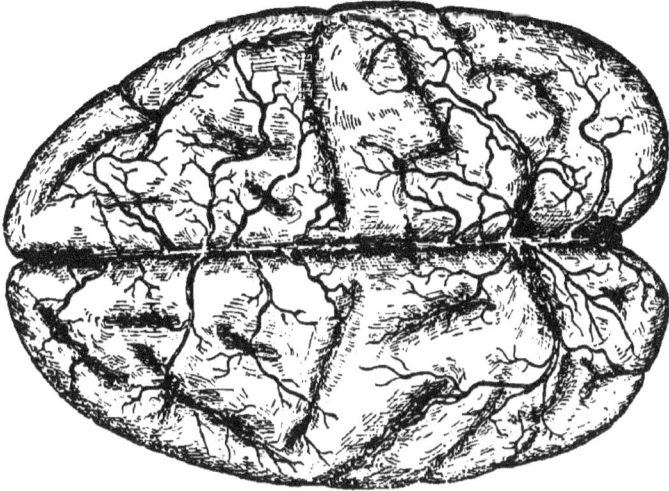

Supra-cerebral veins of the monkey.

FIG. 2.

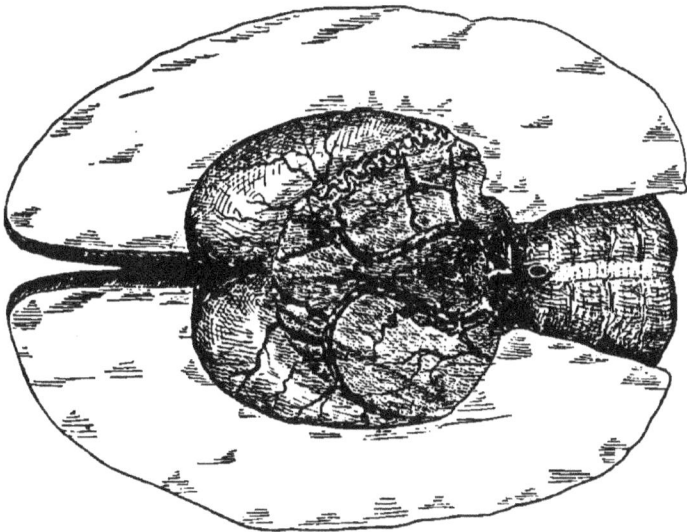

Cœlian veins of the monkey. The basilar is seen on each side, coming up behind the thalamus; that on the right empties directly into Galen's vein, while that on the left ends in the resp. velar. The choroid vein is shown on the right only.

PLATE I.

PLATE II.

FIG. 3.

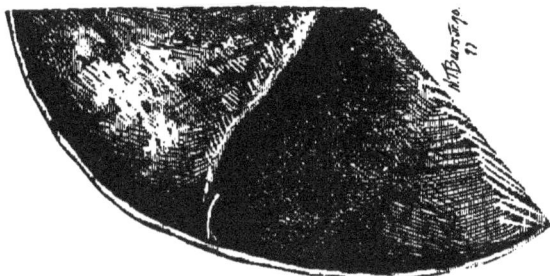

Spheno-temporal emissary in the monkey ; indicated by the white line.

FIG. 4.

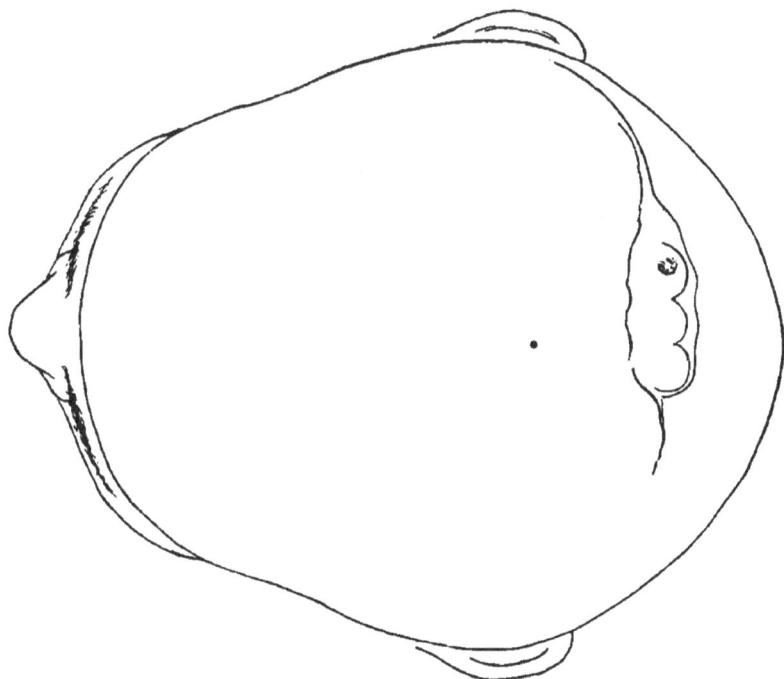

Outline of cranial fissure and depression in the case of old traumatic cephalhydrocele.

www.ingramcontent.com/pod-product-compliance
Lightning Source LLC
Chambersburg PA
CBHW021806190326
41518CB00007B/478